A Journey of Love and Miracles

A Journey of Love and Miracles

Traveling Through Cancer with
the Patient and the Caregiver

Ken and Pat Birt

iUniverse, Inc.
Bloomington

A Journey of Love and Miracles
Traveling Through Cancer with the Patient and the Caregiver

iUniverse books may be ordered through booksellers or by contacting:

iUniverse
1663 Liberty Drive
Bloomington, IN 47403
www.iuniverse.com
1-800-Authors (1-800-288-4677)

ISBN: 978-1-4759-4266-8 (sc)
ISBN: 978-1-4759-4268-2 (hc)
ISBN: 978-1-4759-4267-5 (e)

Library of Congress Control Number: 2012914307

Printed in the United States of America

iUniverse rev. date: 08/07/2012

Dedication

This book is dedicated to John and Dorothy Schneider, Pat's parents, who took the journey, and Sarah Jacobs, our niece, a fellow-traveler on the cancer journey. Also, we include those who have or will travel with us.

This book chronicles the journey of a woman and her caregiver as they face the reality of advanced colorectal cancer head on. There is only so much control physicians and modern medicine have – the sheer will and commitment of a patient plays a large role in the outcome. Pat Birt is evidence of how far determination and strength can take you against the evils of cancer. She never backed down, even when she was given a grave prognosis, and her strict adherence to the recommendations made by her doctors has led to her fantastic state of health. The authors beautifully detail the result of collaboration between a willing patient, a loving caregiver and a multidisciplinary cancer center. While this is an evolving journey, Pat remains an example of the power of love, support and faith.

Dr. Rachna T. Shroff
Assistant Professor, Department of Gastrointestinal (GI) Medical Oncology, Division of Cancer Medicine, The University of Texas MD Anderson Cancer Center, Houston, TX

Table of Contents

Introduction 1

1: A Beginning of the Journey – Bringing Two Together 3

2: Run Like Hell – It's Terminal 13

3: Looking for a New Home Brought New Friends 21

4: The Wedding of Beautiful Memories for a Scared Couple 25

5: More Surgery, More Tumors, Family Tension and Important
Decisions. 31

6: Time to Make Legal Decisions – Time to Live Life 43

7: Hair by Chemo and Now Radiation 49

8: Houston, It's a Go! 55

9: A New Home in Paradise. 59

10: Good News and Now a Honeymoon Cruise. 65

11: Medical Appointments Can Go Awry 71

12: The Impossible Can Be Possible 75

13: The Journey Continues but Never Give Up!. 79

Introduction

●━◆━●

S ome have said this is a story of faith, love and miracles that should be shared with others who face cancer, its prognosis, treatment and aftermath.

But, how does one convey to the cancer patient, primary caregiver, families and friends the experiences of the past twenty-eight months? That is the challenge confronting the authors in writing this book. Will experiences of love and miracles speak to those persons on the cancer journey? Will the things learned by fellow-travelers on the journey be of help? The sole motivation for writing of *A Journey of Love and Miracles: Traveling through Cancer with the Patient and the Caregiver* is to offer hope and support to fellow-travelers. If this book helps just one person, it will have been worth the efforts put forth.

This book is the journey of one couple, complete with fears and difficult decisions but also complete with love, support, joy and miracles. It is chronological and a very personal collection of memories. Sharing the past twenty-eight months, the couple's entire life together, shows what can be accomplished with love for one another and the love of friends and most of all, the love of God. It is hoped that the forty-six suggestions learned and shared in this book will speak to the reader.

It is the honest prayer of the authors that whether a cancer patient or a support person, all will face this insidious disease with hope and courage, that all readers find within this book something that will give the reader the strength to say, "I will never give up!"

Pat Birt

1

◦━◆━◦

A Beginning of the Journey –
Bringing Two Together

K en Birt had moved to Independence, Missouri, leaving his previous home in Oak Ridge, Tennessee, to be near his sister, Barbara, and her extended family. He was recovering from a series of life-changing events. He had retired, attempted adjustment to not working and saw the end of a ten year relationship. And, little did Ken know that his life would be full of more changes and even miracles.

Ken found living alone in a new city, in a new state, in a new region of the country was not all he had hoped for. Without friends and with family members who had their own lives and priorities, he quickly became lonely. Enter, Match.com. Ken's profile on the dating site was simple. He emphasized he was looking for friends and was not a romantic relationship. And, most important, the friends had to live within twenty to thirty miles of Independence.

Pat Baker had also come out of a failed relationship. She lived in Poplar Bluff, Missouri, in the far southeast corner of the State. She worked as Administrative Assistant to the Chief Financial Officer of the regional hospital in Poplar Bluff. She was not a "regular" on match.com. However, on one lonely evening in October, 2009, Pat was looking at members of

Match.com who were residents of Missouri and came across Ken's picture and profile. She was drawn to his pink golf shirt (Pat's favorite color) and his smile. She wrote a short e-mail congratulating Ken on his smile and the thirty-four pound weight loss that he had mentioned in his profile. Ken received the e-mail and thought, "No one ever contacts me on match.com. What is this all about?

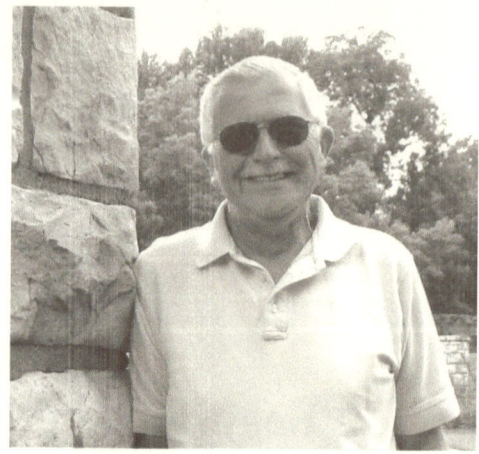

Ken's Match.com Picture

Ken looked at Pat's photo and her profile and responded to Pat in an e-mail, "Where is Poplar Bluff, Missouri?" Regardless of the six hour distance between them, Ken looked at Pat's picture and thought, "She sure is cute."

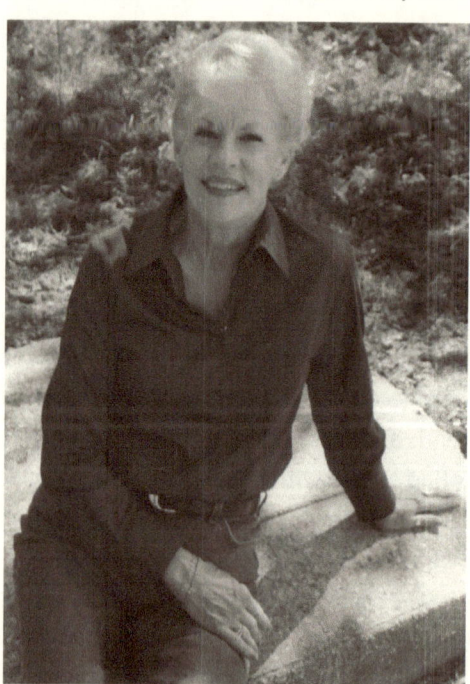

Pat's Match.com Picture

So much for the twenty to thirty mile distance rule!

Ken and Pat spent the remainder of October e-mailing and talking via Yahoo.com on a daily basis. Toward the end of the month, Ken began calling Pat and having lengthy conversations by phone. He learned about Pat's occupation and Pat learned that Ken worked part time in the "Leave No Child Behind Program" administered by a company called Achievia. Ken tutored groups of young elementary-aged children in Math and English and had recently become responsible for several schools, supervising the tutors assigned to those schools. As the days and weeks passed Ken decided, "I need to meet this woman regardless of my distance rule." Pat and Ken began to plan his visit to Poplar Bluff, Missouri.

In early November, 2009, Ken made his first trip to Poplar Bluff. It was a Friday and Pat was working. Ken, an early riser, had left Independence before daylight. He reached Poplar Bluff around Eleven A.M. After looking over the main thoroughfare of the small town and buying a pink rose for Pat, Ken met her at her home during her lunch break. They had a sandwich and Pat returned to work and Ken settled down for a much needed nap. Some things never change!

The weekend was fun. Ken and Pat went to Big Springs, a park a half hour from Poplar Bluff. There is a beautiful river running through the park

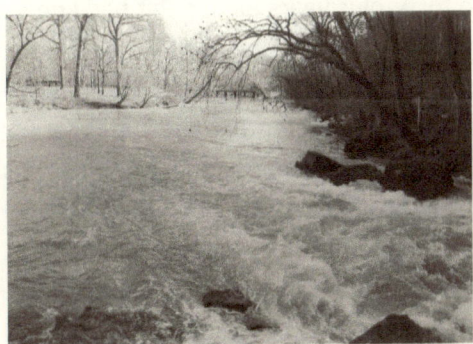

fed by bubbling springs at the base of a rock cliff. Then they drove to Alley Springs and visited another nice park. On the way back to Poplar Bluff, they stopped for ice cream and at a small gift shop. Ken knew of Pat's love of bears and her favorite color, pink, so bought her a small pink stuffed bear.

Big Springs

Before Ken's leaving, Pat told him that her mother, a cousin and his wife, and Pat's half brother and his wife were coming to Poplar Bluff for Thanksgiving and asked, "Could you come for the weekend?" Ken had no plans so decided to make the trip.

On the Tuesday before Thanksgiving, Ken began another trip to Poplar Bluff. Pat had arranged to take the day

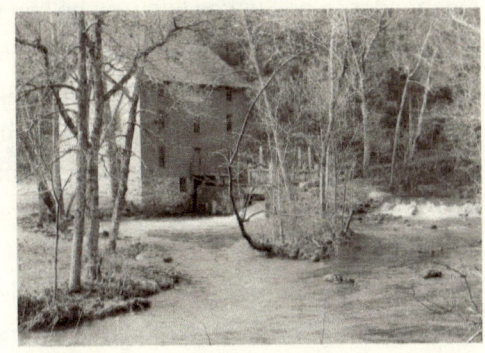

Alley Springs

before Thanksgiving from her job so they both worked together preparing the Thanksgiving meal. Ken offered to peel the potatoes for Pat. Ken peeled a dozen or more potatoes, dropping the peelings into the sink. Then he turned on the garbage disposal. Bad decision. The sink refused to drain and it was obvious that the potato peels had clogged the drain. Ken got a plunger but nothing would clear the clog. This event introduced Ken to another side of Pat. Pat calmly went to her tool chest, found a wrench, got under the sink, loosened and removed the drain pipe, cleared the obstruction (pounds of potato peels) and the problem was solved. "Wow," Ken realized, "There's more to this woman than I thought."

Pat's half brother and his wife arrived mid-Thanksgiving morning. Her brother's name is John and his wife's name is Tammy. Pat had shared the story of John with Ken earlier. It seems that John was the product of a relationship of her father's some forty-plus years earlier. Pat had known of John's existence but had never met him. After her father's death, Pat found a relative of John's mother who contacted John and told him of the sister he never knew he had. John had contacted Pat and they met for the first time. It was exciting for both of them. Pat had no other siblings and John had no idea he had an older half-sister. Pat and her new-found brother seemed happy to have begun a family relationship.

Pat's mother, Dorothy, arrived with Pat's cousin, Gary, and his wife, Terri. Ken was a little nervous about meeting Dorothy and Terri since he had heard Terri was a no-nonsense woman who either liked you or didn't. Fortunately, Ken seemed to pass the test with everyone. Dinner was great and the family had more time really to get to know one another. Ken returned to Independence on Sunday knowing he had to work on Monday.

During the following week, Pat invited Ken to come back to Poplar Bluff for a Physician's Christmas Party sponsored by the hospital. This would be the second weekend in December. Ken accepted. By now, both Ken and Pat knew this relationship was more than casual. Ken, joking, even asked Pat what kind of ring she would like if they got even more serious. Ken thought, "We are in our late 60's. Pat will just want a plain band that will match one for me." WRONG! Pat replied, "A solitaire in a gold setting." Pat now says, "Well, he asked what I wanted and I told him. But, I didn't expect to get it." Did she get it? Read on and see.

Ken made the third trip to Poplar Bluff, helped Pat decide which of three very nice formal dresses to wear and attended the Physician's Party. Ken got a chance to meet many of Pat's co-workers, friends who would mean so much to them over the next year.

During this visit to Poplar Bluff, Ken had decided that he did want to propose to Pat. Ken and Pat drove the two hours to Antonia, Missouri, outside St. Louis, to see Pat's mother. On that trip, Ken asked Pat to go outside while he spoke to Pat's mom. Ken told Dorothy that he was going to propose to Pat. Dorothy seemed happy with that news. Later, Ken invited Pat to come to Independence the week between Christmas and the New Year. Pat accepted and planned to drive to Independence on December 26 after spending Christmas in Antonia, Missouri, with her Mom and Pat's younger son, Bryan. Ken began thinking about proposing during that week and began to look for that solitaire.

Ken's oldest niece, Martha, and her husband Dennis, had a friend who owned a jewelry store. Martha assured Ken that Carolyn, the friend, would make him a wonderful "deal" on the ring. Ken went to the jewelry store and asked to see a solitaire so he could get an idea of the price. Carolyn brought out a beautiful stone. It was perfect. Ken asked the price and almost needed smelling salts. "Can you show me something a little smaller?" Ken asked. Well, as anyone who has first seen the perfect stone can attest, everything else looked small and cheap. Ken bought that first solitaire that he knew Pat would love.

Now, how would Ken propose to Pat? Ken has a sister, Barbara, two nieces and their husbands, and numerous great nieces and great-great nieces in the Kansas City area. After some discussion, everyone thought the proposal ought to happen on December 27, 2009, at the home of Becky and B. J., one of Ken's nieces and her husband. The plan was to have a nice sit down dinner with the whole family in attendance and then Ken would propose after dinner

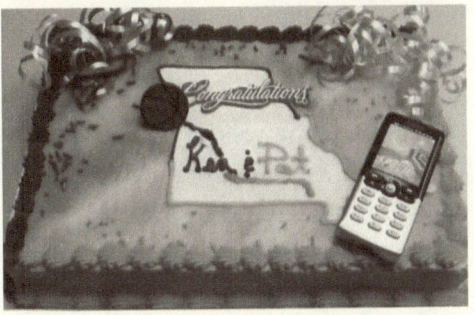

The Engagement Cake

in front of everyone. Ken had an idea for a cake and Becky's daughter, Julia, would arrange it. It would be a sheet cake, half in Duke blue since Ken is a Duke graduate and an avid alum, and half in pink, Pat's favorite color. To emphasize the twenty to thirty mile rule of Ken's, the shape of the state of Missouri would show a line between Independence and Poplar Bluff. At the Independence end, a basketball would represent Ken and at the Poplar Bluff end, a cell phone would represent Pat, since so much of their early sharing had happened by phone. The cake would simply say "Congratulations Ken and Pat."

The day for Pat's arrival in Independence was December 26. The Kansas City area had experienced one of its worst snowfalls in years. Pat's older son, Jeff, lives near Kansas City and is a police lieutenant. He warned Pat, "Mom, it's really bad here. Are you sure you want to come?" Pat was in Antonia and the weather was sunny and pleasant and she said, "Sure, it'll be OK, son." Pat left Antonia and started the four and a half hour drive across the state. About half way, it began to sleet. The sleet was mixed with rain. And then, the snow started falling. Only one lane of I-70 W was open. Pat fell in behind a large truck and just followed. She was afraid to pull off the Interstate to get something to eat or drink or even take a bathroom break for fear of not being able to reenter the highway. Ken and Pat stayed in communication by phone as she made the trip. About four in the afternoon, Pat told Ken she was drawing near his duplex. Ken went to the front door and saw Pat at the base of a long hill leading up to the cul-de-sac on which his duplex sat. On the phone, Pat said, "Ken, I can't get up the hill." Ken said, "Back out and drive to the shopping strip area a block away, park and my neighbor will come in his four-wheel drive truck to get you." Pat nervously backed down the street with cars on both sides, scared she would slide into one. She did make it to the shopping strip and parked. The neighbor in his truck pulled up beside her. Now remember, Pat left beautiful weather. She was in a nice pant suit with dress shoes. The snow was over a foot high. She just passed her bags to the neighbor and slid to his truck. He delivered Pat to Ken's door.

Ken didn't know his neighbors well, having only spoken to them several times sitting on their patios. The neighbors invited Ken and Pat to have dinner with them.

Not being prepared for the amount of snow, the following day Pat took a gift card she had received for Christmas and bought a pair of boots she still refers to as her "logging boots." Living in Missouri, she got a lot of use from them.

The "engagement" party was planned for that evening. The road was clear enough for Pat and Ken to drive to Becky and B. J. Moyers' home. Upon arriving at the Moyer home, Pat was shocked at the number of people. There were over twenty family and friends there for the sit down dinner. Pat met everyone and was a hit with the family. Ken's sister, Barbara, and his niece's husband, Dennis, a policeman in Independence, had to leave to play and sing for a sing-along in a retirement home. But, they promised to be back for dessert. Upon their return, everyone was invited into the living room. Pat thought this strange since the house was huge

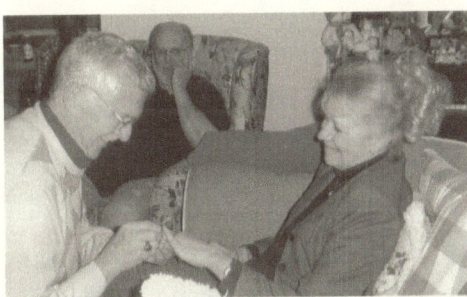

Will You Marry Me?

and the living room relatively small. But, chairs were set up and Pat thought, "Maybe this is a family tradition, having dessert in the living room." Ken invited Pat to sit on a sofa next to him. Then Ken did the strangest thing. He began telling the assembled group how he and Pat had met. It was a rather long and drawn out story. Pat was convinced that Ken was crazy. Then closing the story, Ken said, "Now Pat, the family has met you and you have met the family. It's time to make you an official member." One of Ken's nieces had crawled around behind the sofa where Ken and Pat were sitting and had the ring on a heart-shaped dish. Ken got on his knees and asked Pat, "Will you marry me?" All twenty-plus people applauded. Thankfully, Pat accepted. The only concern the family had was whether

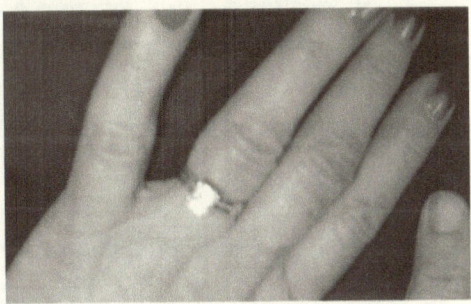

The Solitaire

Ken could get up from his knees. Congratulations flowed for a long time and the cake was brought out and enjoyed. Pat and Ken were engaged.

Over the following days Ken noticed that Pat was experiencing some pain as she got in and out of the car. She excused this by saying that she probably pulled her back lifting her luggage out of the trunk at her mother's. This story satisfied Ken but was something less than the reality. Pat had been suffering pain for a long period of time, but nothing had been uncovered after numerous visits to a number of doctors. (The history of her attempts to find the source of her pain will be covered in a later chapter of this book.)

> *Throughout this book, things that Ken and Pat have learned will be listed as suggestions.*

> *Suggestion #1: It is important to tell those closest to you if you experience any discomfort or symptoms of any kind that concern you. Another person, friend or family, can support and perhaps advise you.*

During earlier conversations, Ken had promised that he'd take Pat on a cruise for their honeymoon since Pat had never been on a cruise. The day after the engagement, Ken took Pat to AAA where they booked a one-week cruise to the Caribbean in May, thinking they'd marry in that month. Pat was flabbergasted. So much had happened in a relatively short period of time and Pat was overwhelmed.

> *Suggestion #2: It is always a good idea when planning a cruise or trip where trip insurance is available to pay the small amount for that. In the event of sickness or emergency, the insurance will save you from the lost investment.*

New Year's Eve came and Ken had made reservations at his favorite restaurant, Yia Yia's in Overland Park, Kansas just outside Kansas City. They had no plans after dinner so decided to go to a casino where Pat played a slot machine near Ken. They were both dressed to the hilt for New Year's Eve. A lady playing next to Pat said, "Is that your man down the line here?"

Pat replied, "Yes, it is." The woman continued, "You are a striking couple." That's a comment they have often heard and continue to hear. Pat beams every time.

Two days later, Pat returned to Poplar Bluff ready to show off "the rock" to everyone. Pat worked with a

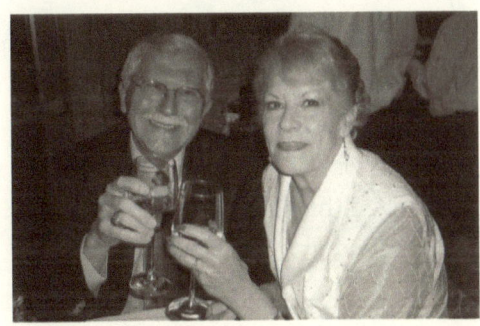

New Year's at Yia Yia's

young woman, Stacy. The first morning Pat approached Stacy, held out her left hand and asked, "How do you like my new finger nail polish?" Stacy looked and replied, "Yes, it's nice" and walked away. A minute later she stopped in her tracks and said, "My God!" She had just realized that Pat was wearing an engagement ring. Everyone in Pat's office was thrilled for her.

The snow that had hit the Kansas City area returned the first week of January, 2010 with a vengeance. Ken was not tutoring but was substituting and also managing the tutors in the school assigned to him. Since the weather caused school closures he was getting no work. Pat and Ken had decided on Ken's joining Pat in Poplar Bluff in May when school was out. Because of no work, Ken thought, "My lease on the duplex ends in February. By moving earlier, I can actually save more money than I make. I can join Pat earlier." Ken and Pat began to plan the move. It was set for February 14. Ken began packing boxes and storing them in his garage. He arranged the rental of a truck and Pat contacted some friends to travel with her to Independence and help load the truck. On Friday, February 13, they arrived, loaded the truck and left for Poplar Bluff the morning of the 14th. They began unloading the truck on Sunday, February 15.

Suggestion #3: Listen to your inner-self. Sometimes a change of plans might be exactly what God directs. God works in marvelous ways and Ken and Pat believe

He does communicate with you and directs you in the correct path.

Ken had made the move to Poplar Bluff. Again, little did they know that the next week would further impact their lives as nothing in the past ever had.

What were the climatic events of the week of February 16, 2010, that so changed their lives?

2

◦—◆—◦

Run Like Hell – It's Terminal

Pat had been experiencing significant pain in her abdomen area for almost two years. This discomfort was something Ken had not learned of until recently. Her first complaint was to her family doctor. He initially prescribed a colonoscopy, which showed nothing. When the pain persisted, he referred Pat to Dr. Kean Griffith of Ozark Medical Management, a part of the Poplar Bluff Regional Medical Center. Dr. Griffith performed another colonoscopy, again showing nothing. Dr. Griffith referred her to a doctor in Cape Girardeau, Missouri, where Pat underwent a capsule endoscopy, an eight hour procedure, which also showed nothing. Pat had also gone to her OB/GYN for an annual pap smear. The doctor thought that Pat had an inflamed colon and prescribed an antibiotic for her. Still, there was no relief. Following that, Pat had a lower bowel scan which showed nothing. Pat returned to Dr. Griffith and asked what should be done next. The response was, "There is no NEXT." Pat felt that she was being viewed as a hypochondriac. But, the pain still persisted.

> *Suggestion #4: When you experience a continuing health issue that can't be diagnosed, it is time for you to have an advocate with you, a person who will ask the hard questions and make sure the medical personnel use every*

option at their disposal. In Pat's case, many laypersons would have thought, "Why not a CAT Scan?"

One night when Pat turned over in bed, she felt a sharp pain and actually could feel a lump in her abdomen. She went to her family doctor and he thought it was an impacted bowel. At Kneibert Clinic in Poplar Bluff, she had X-rays that didn't produce any new results. Pat's family physician referred her back to Dr. Griffith.

It was Monday, February 16, 2010, the day after Ken's move to Poplar Bluff. Dr. Griffith had scheduled a consultation with Pat that led her to another colonoscopy on Tuesday. During that procedure, technician Angie Taylor, working with Dr. Griffith, suggested that the doctor look into a recessed opening that appeared to be a hole in the colon; it was visible on the screen. Dr. Griffith double-checked and discovered that there was a tumor, not just a small tumor, but one the size of a grapefruit. Why had the several colonoscopies not shown it? It was attached to the outside of the colon. Surgery was set for the next day.

The home garage was full of boxes. Ken had not even begun to unpack. Now Pat was in the hospital.

Ken and Pat believe with no doubt that this was the first of a number of medical miracles in their life together. Ken had originally planned on moving to join Pat in May. The move was rescheduled to February just two days before Pat had serious surgery. Pat had no family in Poplar Bluff and Ken provided the support system she needed during this first event. Was this a coincidence or was it God working in His sometime mysterious way to care for His children?

Pat's surgery was major. Her pancreas, liver and stomach were scraped for tissue samples for biopsy. Ten lymph nodes were removed. Two feet of her colon were removed for examination. Of the ten lymph nodes, four were cancerous. The grapefruit-sized tumor was malignant. Fortunately, the tissue samples from the pancreas, liver and stomach were benign.

Upon Pat's returning to her room, people who worked with Pat at the hospital started coming by to check on her. They were understanding of her need for rest and only wished her the best. However, one of Pat's acquaintances, a lady who seemed to think she should have the initials

MD after her name, decided it was her responsibility to approach the nurses' station and give the nurses direction. The neighbor had only met Ken once but Ken made it very clear that if help was needed for Pat, he would see she got it. Ken also requested that friends and neighbors not tell Pat any cancer stories, either good or bad. During his professional years in the ministry, Ken had learned that every patient needs an advocate and that was now his responsibility. A positive attitude from everyone was the number one requirement.

> *Suggestion #5: Encourage friends and relatives to be positive with the patient. One person needs to be the patient's advocate. That person must be a strong advocate. Having a number of people sharing their cancer stories with the patient can be very disturbing. Friends should do the loving things that friends do, bring dinners, magazines and books, offer to clean the house or run errands. The common statement made by friends is "Let me know if you need anything!" Supporters, don't wait to be asked. Just do those small things that will mean so much to the patient and his or her family.*

A hour or so after surgery, Dr. Griffith came by the room. He checked on Pat's vital signs and dressings and went out into the hall.

Ken followed him and asked, "Dr. Griffith, what is the prognosis."

Dr. Griffith responded, "Not good at all."

Ken asked, "Not good, as in terminal?"

Dr. Griffith responded "Yes, it's stage four colon cancer and my experience has been that the patient has a one in four chance of survival."

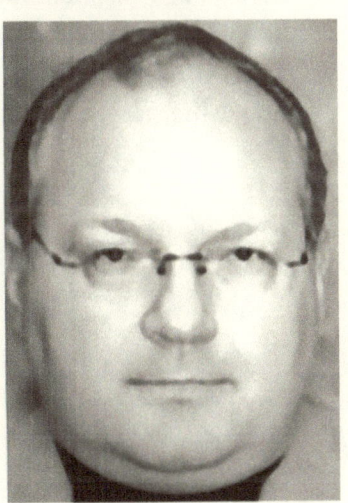

Dr. Kean Griffith

Ken asked, "What is the life expectancy?"

Dr. Griffith responded, "Probably a year."

Ken was devastated. Ken thought, "Our life is just starting. Should I tell Pat or not?" He decided that since Pat was still under the influence of the medication, he'd let Dr. Griffith talk to her the next morning. However, later that evening, Pat knew something was troubling Ken and asked him what it was. Ken sat, held Pat's hand and told her what Dr. Griffith had said. They cried together. At that moment, who should come in but Pat's supervisor, Mark Johnson, the Chief Financial Officer of the hospital and his partner, Scott Bradshaw, with a get well card in hand. What a wonderful visit that was! It was followed shortly by a visit from Lisa Carda, the wife of the Chief Executive Officer of the hospital, Greg Carda, who sat on the side of Pat's bed and showed such love and concern. Later, Greg paid his own visit. Mark, Scott, Greg and Lisa continue to be great friends today.

Pat remained in the hospital for ten days. Her son Bryan brought her mother to visit. Looking for a cup of coffee, Bryan and Ken went to the cafeteria. Outside, as they walked down the hall, Bryan said, "Ken, I'd run like hell if I was you." Ken assured Bryan he had no intention of running. Bryan later said, "I was just testing you." Pat's older son, Jeff, drove from Excelsior Springs, Missouri, and spent a day visiting.

During Pat's hospitalization another interesting event took place that they consider a miracle. Pat had chosen to take out Aflac Cancer Insurance years earlier. The hospital had allowed it as a payroll deduction but had recently withdrawn the deduction option and chosen another company.

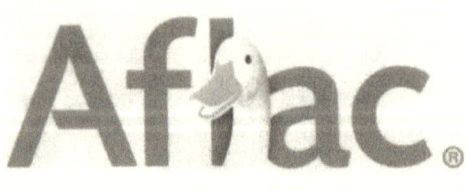

If Pat wanted Aflac, she'd have to fill out forms and have it transferred so that she'd be paying it personally. During one of Ken's previous visits, Pat and Ken had

Aflac Logo

discussed whether Aflac was needed or not. Ken had always been advised that it wasn't a wise investment so they were thinking whether to continue the insurance or not. With all that was happening, they had just forgotten to make the decision. Ken had left the hospital and gone to the house and was sitting at Pat's desktop computer. He looked at a stack of mail and noticed the form from Aflac that had to be sent in for continuation. Ken looked at the due date and it was just two days off. He almost panicked. He quickly filled out the form, put down his Visa Card number, stamped the envelope and rushed to the post office. Was it a coincidence that Ken was at that desk on that day? Ken and Pat don't think so because the Aflac insurance has been a life-saver making it possible for them financially to handle much of this journey. Ken's negative attitude about cancer insurance has changed.

> *Suggestion #6: Ken had always thought cancer insurance was a waste of money. Not so! It is a small price to pay for the financial help the insurance can offer. Health Insurance should be kept up to date and should cover prescription costs. But where will the money come from that will pay for costs not covered by health insurance? Aflac is one provider of cancer insurance. There are others. It IS a good investment.*

During Pat's second or third day in the hospital, she was visited by Dr. Ray Peters, the chemo oncologist with the hospital. It was determined that Pat would have to recover from the surgery prior to chemo. A PET scan was scheduled for March 10 as well as a port (a device through which to draw blood or deliver the chemo cocktail) being implanted by Dr. Griffith on March 17. The chemo was scheduled to begin March 18, 2010.

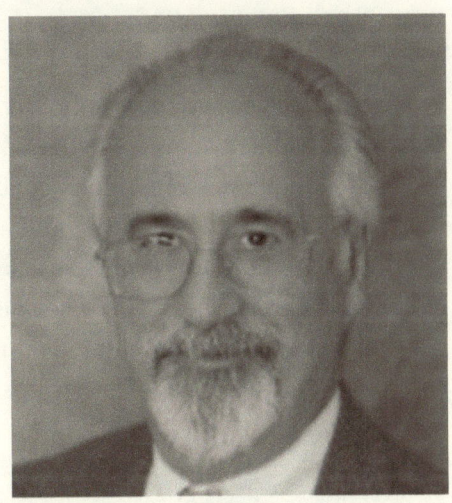

Dr. Ray Peters

Ken and Pat discussed the date for their wedding and the honeymoon cruise. Pat wanted to be at her best for both and it was decided to postpone the wedding from early May and cancel the cruise. Fortunately, Ken had taken out cancellation insurance so that no money was lost in the cruise cancellation. The date for the wedding was put on hold.

On March 18, the chemo began. Dr. Peters also wanted Pat to take Xeloda, an oral chemo drug. While Pat was going through the first chemo treatment, Ken offered to take the Xeloda prescription to the Kroger Pharmacy and have it filled. At Kroger, Ken was told that Pat's insurance would not pay for Xeloda. Ken simply said, "That's OK. We'll work that out. Just fill the prescription." They replied, "Do you know that it will be $1,200?" Ken was shocked and replied, "Let's put that off until we can talk to the doctor." Ken returned to the Ambulatory Infusion Center and passed the news to Pat. They then, with Dr. Peters' assistance, made inquiries into other sources for Xeloda. Sometime later, they were able to purchase the oral chemo drug through a mail order prescription company with all costs covered by Pat's insurance.

> **Suggestion #7: In the event that a patient's insurance does not cover a medication, talk to the doctor and his or her staff. They can be of tremendous help and can often find a solution.**

Pat was to receive her chemotherapy every two weeks. In order to keep Pat's platelet numbers under control, it was necessary for her to receive a shot in the stomach on her visits for chemo. (Platelets are small cell fragments produced in the bone marrow that help the blood clot.) Although the shots are never pleasant, Pat withstood them with little discomfort. The journey toward healing had begun, but they had no idea what that journey would entail. Ken never doubted that Pat would be cured and Pat rarely gave up her positive attitude. There was just too much to live for.

> **Suggestion #8: The patient should have an advocate, usually a family member or a friend. That person should be with the patient on every treatment and every doctor's visit. The advocate can ask the hard questions, ask for an explanation when something is not understood**

and watch for consistency in the treatments. If a step seems to be left out, the patient or advocate should ask why. Doctors and treatment centers do make mistakes, so ask!

From the time of Ken's first visit to Poplar Bluff, he and Pat had been attending First United Methodist Church. Ken, being a retired minister, spent time with the Senior Pastor, The Reverend Charles Buck. Pastor Buck had a wonderful gift of ministry to those who were undergoing difficult times. Not a day passed that he did not visit Pat in the hospital, sharing encouragement and prayer. This ministry became very important in both Ken's and Pat's spiritual lives.

Pastor Charles Buck

In addition to Charles' ministry, Ken and Pat had become active in the Phoenix Sunday School Class. Pat already knew many of the class. Some were doctors at the hospital. Others were people Pat had met during her residency in Poplar Bluff. Ken and Pat weren't members of the church yet, but were taken into the class with open arms. When Pat left the hospital, the class prepared meals and delivered them to their home. Ken and Pat will always hold those people close to their hearts. They definitely represented what Christian discipleship is all about.

Suggestion #9: If you are a person of faith, make your congregation and especially your pastor, priest or religious leader fully aware of your condition. The pastor will visit, listen and offer prayer. The small groups within the congregation will also bring comfort and offer their help. Accept that help! Make them a part of your team!

Pat was under a doctor's care and doing reasonably well. Chemo left her drained for a couple days after each treatment, but she suffered through like the trooper she is. Other priorities in the Birts' lives could be addressed now. What were they and how did they proceed with the shadow of cancer always present?

3

Looking for a New Home Brought New Friends

One of the concerns for the Birts during the early days of their journey and marriage was Pat's mother. Dorothy was 87 years old. She still lived in the house she called home for over 51 years. Bryan, Pat's 40 year old son, lived with Pat's mom, but he was single and had a life of his own. Pat and Ken knew that they could not be sure of their availability to care for her mother if the need arose. When Pat tried to talk to her mother about other options, Dorothy's reply was always, "I'll cross that bridge when I come to it." She still drove on local errands, but that was a concern to Pat and Ken as well. So, in March 2010, they decided that they would look at some options for Dorothy in the event she might reconsider going to an assisted living facility. Ken's sister, Barbara, was very happy in The Carlyle, a very nice facility in Lee's Summit, Missouri. Ken did

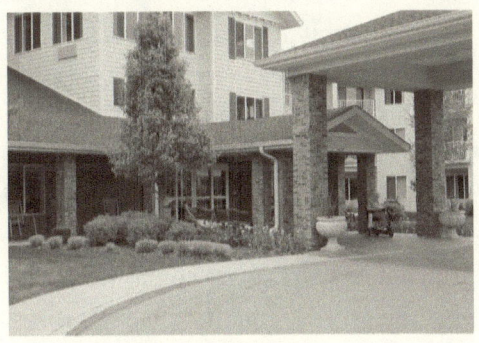

The Orchid Terrace

research and learned that a sister-facility, The Orchid Terrace, was in St. Louis. He made a phone call to them and set an appointment to visit and tour.

> *Suggestion 10: If the patient or immediate family has a senior parent, assure that person is taken care of and that minimal help will be needed by the patient or his or her immediate family. Make sure the senior parent's affairs are in order in the event of a death or serious illness. The patient and immediate family have a full plate and shouldn't have to worry about caring for an aging parent's affairs. Sometimes the most caring thing is to plan ahead.*

During this time Pat was still undergoing her chemotherapy and feeling reasonably well. One Friday, Ken and Pat drove the two hours to St. Louis to

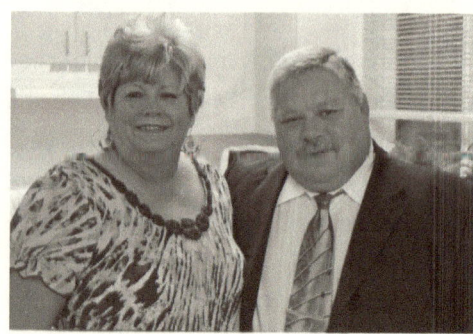

Linda and Lonnie Orsborn

The Orchid Terrace. They were supposed to meet with one of the Assistant Managers, but when they arrived, those assistants were scheduled to leave for their weekend off. Instead, Ken and Pat met with the Managers, Linda and Lonnie Orsborn. They were a delightful couple and Ken and Pat were shown all the apartment options. They even liked the facility so much that they wondered if this option might be best for them, not knowing Pat's future and their ability to keep up with the responsibility of a home and yard. Ken and Pat were invited to lunch at The Orchid Terrace with the Orsborns and that started a friendship that lasted throughout their residency in Missouri.

Pat and Ken had not confirmed a date for their wedding. Just too much else was on their minds. Ken had made a trip to Bahama, North Carolina, to visit his friends of thirty-seven years, Dr. F. Belton Joyner, Jr. and his wife, Toni. Ken had been Belton's Assistant in Ministry in Mebane, North Carolina, from 1975 through 1978 while Ken was in seminary at Duke University. Their friendship had continued through the years. Ken and Pat knew that they wanted Belton to perform the wedding ceremony. Ken and Pat had even considered just having a simple service in a park in nearby Durham with only Belton, Toni, a witness and Ken and Pat in attendance. On Ken's trip, he and Belton looked at several outdoor venues for the wedding.

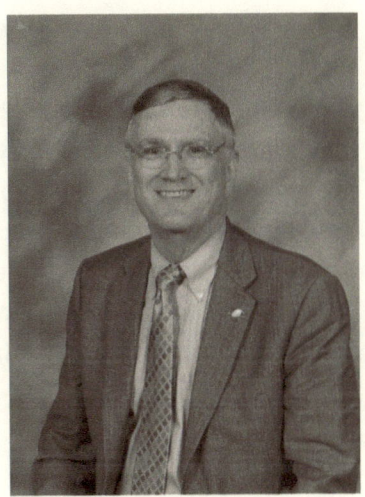

Dr. F. Belton Joyner, Jr.

Suggestion #11: The caretaker needs to have an outlet for their frustrations, physical and psychological needs. The caretaker is the forgotten victim of cancer. Friends, a minister or a caregiver's group can fill this need. However, if the caregiver leaves the home for any length of time, make sure the patient has the care and support they need in the primary caregiver's absence.

While visiting Lonnie and Linda at The Orchid Terrace, Linda asked Pat, "Where are you going to get married?" Pat told Linda of their current thoughts. Linda said, "Oh no, why don't you get married right here? The residents have never had a wedding here and they'd love it." Pat responded that she just didn't think she was up to the planning and work that would have to go into it. Linda said, "Don't worry, Pat, I'll take care of all of that."

Suggestion #12: Don't postpone major events if the patient is well enough to participate. Allow friends to help with the planning and carrying out the event. Friends want to do this. Let them!

Pat was feeling amazingly well. By June, she had completed six chemo sessions and was able to take a break from treatment. So, the wedding was set for Saturday, June 19, 2010. Belton would fly from North Carolina to officiate. Ken's friend of forty years, Alan Galumbeck, would drive from Atlanta, Georgia, to be Ken's best man. Kathy Schworm, Pat's daughter, would fly from Florida and serve as Pat's matron of honor. Ken's sister, Barbara, would sing. How does a wedding impact the lives of cancer patients and their caregivers? Why would they include the following story in their journey to defeat the dreaded disease?

4

• ◆ •

The Wedding of Beautiful
Memories for a Scared Couple

P at and Ken began to buy small items for the wedding: two joined hearts, with white flowers and beads to top off the cake, pink rose petals for the flower girl to drop, as well as other items. Pat has no siblings other than John, her younger half brother, but she has more cousins than Ken can count (or remember the names of). One of those cousins, Donna Schneider, was employed by a party rental firm and Ken and Pat arranged for a beautiful arch, kneeling rail and holder for the unity candles.

Linda Orsborn went straight to work. She made arrangements for a cake, a champagne fountain and, a week before the wedding, began decorating the winding stair railing and balcony railings with greenery and artificial flowers. She also hung paper bells from the chandeliers in the room where the wedding would take place. She took mints that Pat and Ken had purchased and wrapped the heart shaped boxes in white netting and tied them with a bow as well as placing a small card on each, noting it was celebration of Pat and Ken's wedding.

The normal dinner time for the residents was 6:00 pm. Lonnie and Linda moved it to 5:30 so dinner could be served and the dining room cleared and set up for the service at 7:00 pm. Belton made arrangement for his flight so he'd arrive the day before the wedding and Alan arranged his drive to arrive on Friday also. Linda said, "Don't worry about lodging for Belton, Kathy or yourselves. We have two furnished apartments for you and Belton. And, we can set up a rollaway bed in an empty apartment for Kathy." Alan had made arrangements for a hotel nearby. Arrangements were also confirmed for a hotel room for Barbara, Ken's sister, who would drive from the Kansas City area. Ken and Pat would pick up Dorothy, Pat's mother, in Antonia, only a thirty minute drive away.

One wedding concern was who would play the necessary wedding music. Ken had been in contact with a United Methodist church in St. Louis in the event he and Pat moved there. He e-mailed the Associate Pastor for ideas. That pastor suggested the Music Director of the church, Jim Theilker, who readily agreed to play. The Orchid Terrace had a beautiful electronic baby grand piano that would fill the need. It was moved into the dining room.

The day of the wedding had arrived. Pat had not received chemo for several weeks and felt good. Linda had arranged a nice lunch in the private dining room for the wedding party. Further decorating continued with many of the Orchid Terrace staff helping. Greenery and flowers were woven into the arch. Everyone arrived on time, including Steve and Rose Anne Bell, parishioners from Ken's last church in Oak Ridge, Tennessee.

A couple of hours prior to the wedding dinner, Barbara arrived to rehearse with Jim, the pianist/organist. She was to sing *The Lord's Prayer*

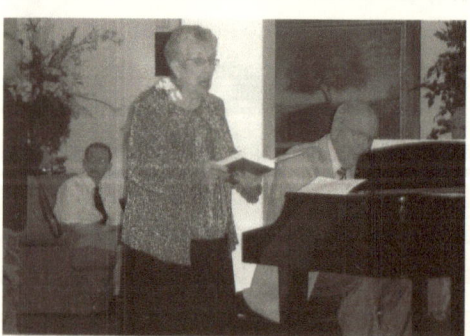

Barbara Singing *The Lord's Prayer*

during Communion as well as a favorite hymn of Ken's, *Be Thou My Vision*, before the service. Everyone was decorating when Barbara began singing *The Lord's Prayer* in practice. They all stopped what they were doing and were mesmerized by Barbara's singing. There were even a few tears shed. Even though Barbara was 79 years old, her voice was as beautiful and strong as it ever had been.

Dinner time came. Linda had arranged a wonderful dinner for forty guests as well as the residents of The Orchid Terrace.

Ken and Pat dressed in semi-formal outfits for the dinner. They would later change into more formal clothes for the wedding.

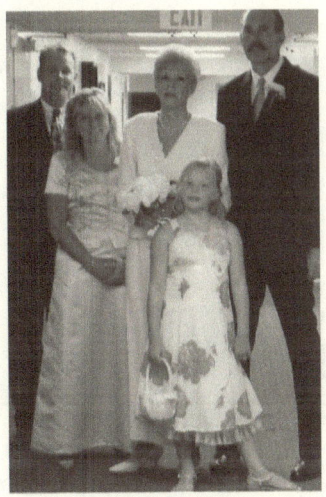

Bryan, Kathy, Pat, Kaylee and Jeff before the Service

Kaylee Cowden, the granddaughter of Pat's friend, Debbie Doiron, served as the flower girl and spread the pink rose petals on the stairway before Pat, escorted by her two sons, Bryan and Jeff, came down the stairs. Bry-

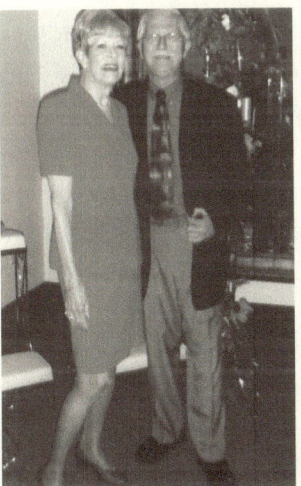

Pat and Ken Dressed for Wedding Dinner

an, always the comedian, asked his mother, "What do I do?" Pat said, "Don't let me fall." Bryan

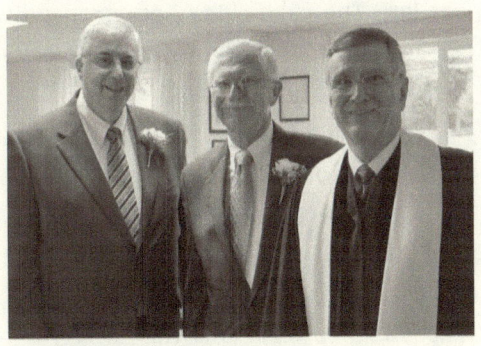

Alan, Ken and Belton Prior to Service

replied, "Do your feet have to touch the floor?"

Time came for the service and it was perfect. Pat's Mom had asked Pat why she wanted a larger wedding at her age. After the service Dorothy commented that it was the most beautiful wedding she had ever attended. Forty-five of the residents and forty of the Birts' guests were present. The

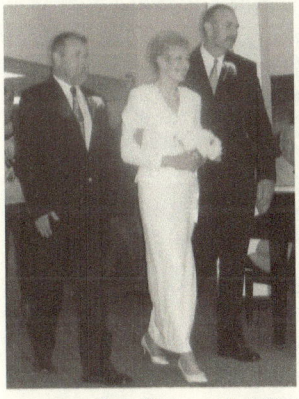

Bryan and Jeff Escorting Pat

room was full. Following Kaylee, the flower girl, Pat's beautiful daughter came down the stairs, followed by Jeff and Bryan, escorting their mother.

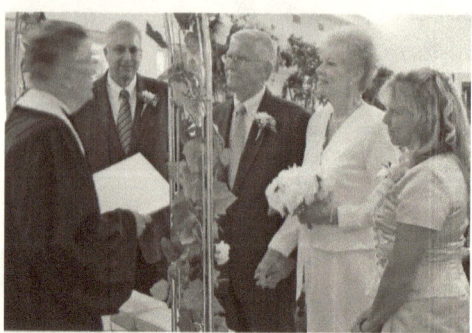

Belton, Alan, Ken, Pat and
Kathy During the Vows

During the service, Belton shared the story behind the ring Pat gave Ken. It had been Pat's grandmother's and had passed on to Pat's father who had worn it as his wedding band. Pat wanted Ken to have it as his wedding band if he didn't mind not getting a new ring. Ken was thrilled to have the ring with such strong tradition. Communion was part of the service. Pat, Ken, Belton and Rose Anne Bell served.

After the service, a very nice reception was held. Ken and Pat were amazed at how much the residents loved the champagne. Not a drop was left. The cake Linda had arranged was perfect. Pat was somewhat concerned when she heard it was to be white with beige trim. It could not have been more beautiful.

The final amazing thing was that Lonnie and Linda would not let Ken and Pat pay for a thing. The rooms, the luncheon, the dinner, the reception and all the decorating was their gift. What a blessing this was to Pat and Ken! It was far more than they could have ever afforded or expected. Was this yet another miracle in their journey as husband and wife? Just how

long would Pat have for "the rest of her life?" In the back of their minds were still the words of Dr. Griffith: "One in four chance of living and maybe only a year."

One additional note. Ken and Pat still hadn't planned a honeymoon. Pat's Mom and Belton were huge St. Louis

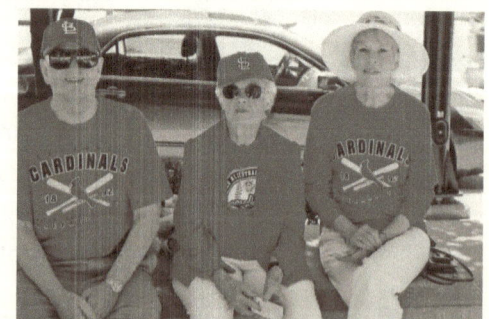

Belton, Pat's Mom, Dorothy and
Pat at Cardinal's Game

Cardinals baseball fans. Pat and Ken's honeymoon? An afternoon Cardinals game with their minister and Ken's new mother-in-law in one hundred and four degree heat. But, they'll never forget it. Never!

Suggestion 13: Be sure that all precautions are taken if the patient is to be in extreme hot weather. Chemo does impact the body's chemistry. Hats and long sleeves should be worn to fend off the heat and, if necessary, the patient should be settled in as a cool a spot as possible.

Now, the reader might ask, "Why a full chapter on your wedding?" The answer is simple. When one is faced with a tragedy as frightening as cancer, it is important to continue to live life with all the gusto possible. Ken has since stated, "We would have been married if I would have had to wheel Pat down the aisle in a hospital bed."

Suggestion 14: Continue to live life with all the gusto possible. Everyone has a "bucket list" whether it is written or not. Live life! Start living those dreams from the patient's bucket list. Make memories!

Ken's and Pat's wedding was just one of many examples of God's love. He put them together at a time that was vital for both of them. Their marriage was their response to His love. They anticipated not only a marriage but a long, happy and faithful life together. Why did the marriage carry with it the possibility that it might be short? Had Ken and Pat defeated the dreaded "C" or was the journey still in its early stages? Were more miracles in store, or had they used up their share? Jim Valvano's words spoke to them yet again. "Don't give up. Never give up!"

5

$\bullet\!-\!\blacklozenge\!-\!\bullet$

More Surgery, More Tumors, Family Tension and Important Decisions

P at's treatments continued. Although she experienced some sickness from the chemotherapy, it only last a few days and then she was fine. In June, 2010, they made a trip to Atlanta, Georgia, to visit Alan Galum-beck, the best man in their wedding. Alan was instrumental in starting the Weather Channel, had retired and lived in the Buckhead section of Atlanta in a penthouse on the sixteenth floor. It was a good trip and Ken, Pat and Alan went to see the Georgia Aquarium. Pat must have felt

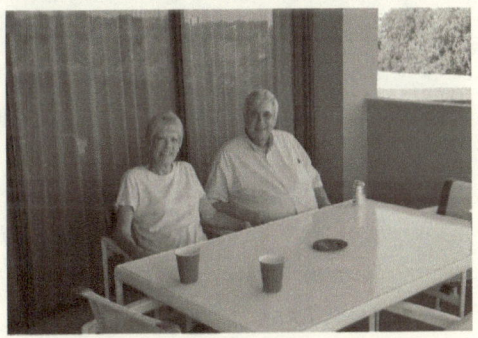
Pat and Alan on Alan's Balcony

pretty good because she asked Alan to rent a carpet shampoo machine and she cleaned his bathrooms and shampooed his carpeting and cleaned the sandstone tile.

Pat had another PET scan in late July, 2010. Another growth that had metastasized from the colon was found on the chest wall. More surgery was required and was performed on August 2, 2010. Dr. Stanley Ziomek, a cardio thoracic surgeon, performed the surgery. Pat has diabetes and led a support group for four years; Dr. Ziomek had been a guest speaker several times. He was known by both Pat and Ken. After a biopsy was obtained by an incision in the throat area, the lemon-sized growth was removed through a cut under her right arm and rib cage and half way up her back. This surgery was far more difficult than previous procedures for Pat. At one point her lung collapsed and

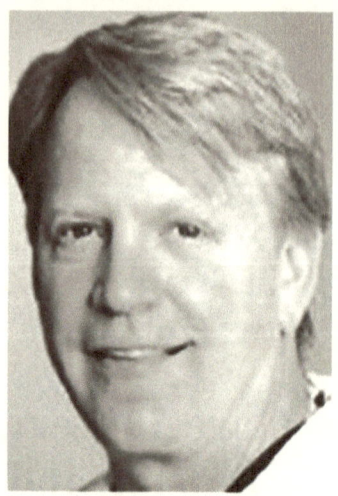

Dr. Stanley Ziomek

she had to be put into ICU. As part of Pat's treatment, Dr. Ziomek's physician assistant, Carla, plunged talc into the drain tube. Thinking this was a simple procedure, Ken sat near the bed and watch. The procedure was far from simple. Ken saw Pat in more pain than he had ever witnessed before and Pat agreed, saying it was the worst pain she had ever experienced including child birth.

During this surgery and its aftermath, Pat reached the lowest point she had experienced since the first diagnosis. Thanks to The Reverend Charles Buck, the Birts' pastor, Pat found the comfort she needed. As Charles said, "Sometimes you just have to reach bottom to start the journey up."

> *Suggestion #15: Patients, share your down times with your family, your caregiver and your spiritual support person. If you are a private person, get over it! They want to help. Let them do that!*

While Pat was in the ICU, a very unfortunate event occurred. Patients and families should understand that having a loved one with cancer is very stressful. Pat's half-brother, John, along with his wife, Tammy, and Pat's mother, were visiting. They had left the ICU room so that Pat could be bathed. Ken approached them and said, "She'll be alright. As soon as this lung issue is resolved, she'll be back in her own room and then home." John reacted by saying, "You don't know what will happen. You have no idea." In defense, Ken said, "John, I am her husband. I will be with her every minute." John in anger walked to within inches of Ken and spoke very loudly, "You aren't S***!" and then repeated it two more times. Ken was furious; a nurse came over and warned both John and Ken that if they didn't stop, she'd call security. Ken separated himself from the others. John, his wife, and Pat's mother left the hospital for home. John was stressed as was Ken. Later, John apologized and admitted that Ken had been a tremendous help to Pat and that he realized that now. His step-father had been diagnosed with anal cancer and saw how devastating the lack of support can be. Although that apology took awhile coming, John and Ken are best buddies now.

> *Suggestion #16: Remember, caregivers, family and friends are all under a great amount of stress. Cancer impacts everyone. Be patient with each other. Any serious illness is a time for family togetherness. Be a family. The patients don't need the stress of worrying about those they love battling over their illness.*

This hospitalization lasted for sixteen days. During this time in the hospital a number of things happened. First, all of Pat's sick days, vacation days and FMLA (Family Medical Leave Act) days had been exhausted. Poplar Bluff Regional Medical Center had no choice but to terminate her employment. The termination meant that Ken had to go to the Social Security Office and arrange for her Medicare Part B. Ken had an insurance agent in Kansas City whom he called to sign Pat up for supplemental insurance. The Agent, Laurie Fields, also arranged for a prescription insurance policy for Pat.

> *Suggestion #17: Make sure that all facts related to the patient's employment and insurance coverage are known to family as well as the primary caregiver. Don't be caught unaware that insurance is about to be*

canceled or that income will cease. Be prepared! Have an insurance agent whom you know well and trust.

Ken and Pat's home had been on the market prior to Pat's hospitalization. The house sold a day or so before Pat was hospitalized. Now, papers had to be signed and Pat was in the hospital. Ken made numerous trips back and forth between the hospital and the real estate office handling this.

Suggestion #18: Can the patient and family care for the home in which the patient lives? Can the family take care of the inside as well as the outside of the house? Is it time to downsize to save labor for the patient and family? These are good questions to ask.

Since the house had sold, it was necessary for Ken to find another place for them to live. Here is where another unusual event happened. Miracle? Maybe! Ken had a real aversion to the Poplar Bluff newspaper. He never read it. In the hospital room, Pat had been given that newspaper. Totally bored with nothing else to do, Ken picked up the paper. In it was an ad for a duplex that sounded perfect for them. Ken called the owner, set an appointment and went to see the duplex. It was indeed perfect. On one of Pat's Mom's visits, Ken took her to see it and took pictures to show Pat. The lease was signed without Pat ever seeing the duplex in person. It served as their home for the next year.

Now, Ken had to arrange a move. He went to a U-Haul rental place, a part of a convenience store. He explained to the clerk that his wife was in the hospital, a cancer patient, and he needed to arrange the rental of a truck. The clerk had a line of people waiting and asked if Ken could hold for a few minutes. Ken went and sat in a chair next to a rather scruffy looking young man. The young man looked at Ken and said, "Your wife is in the hospital and you're going to move?" Ken responded, "Yes." The man said, "I might be able to get a few people together to help you." Ken thought, "Hmmmm, this guy probably needs to make some money." Then the young man reached in his pocket and produced a business card. He was the Youth Minister of a church. The following week, the day after Pat was released from the hospital, the young man, his wife, two other adults and 4 youth came to the house and worked all day packing boxes. Now, what are the odds of Ken being in that convenience store at the exact same time as the young youth minister? Is that coincidence? Is that a gift from God? Is that a miracle?

Suggestion #19: Be open to other's offers to help. It's so easy to say, "Thank you, but we have it covered." Even strangers can often help. With security always in mind, allow strangers to become friends. They will be blessed and so will you.

It was time for the move from the three bedroom home in Poplar Bluff to a two bedroom duplex seven miles outside of town. Prior to Pat's leaving the hospital, a number of her friends came with SUV's, trailers and pickups to help Ken move enough furniture to allow Pat to stay comfortably in the new dwelling and avoid the organized chaos of the major move.

On August 21, Ken, with friends, executed the major move and within a few days of Ken's lugging boxes and Pat's opening them, everything was unpacked and in place. They had a new home and Pat was pleased with the choice Ken had made.

A week after the move, a huge garage sale was held at the sold house. Each room was set up individually containing specific items. Linens, curtains, towels and bathroom items were in one room. Kitchen items were in another. Electronics were in one of the bedrooms. Again, a number of friends came to help, even Patsy, a friend from Florida. Pat's supervisor, Mark Johnson, the Chief Financial Officer of the hospital, came also. He seemed to have a great time hawking all the tools and garage items. He'd come to Ken and whisper, "Ken, can you answer a question? I think I've got a hot one!" After the garage sale, the house was cleaned with the help of friends and the move could be considered complete.

Suggestion #20: This fact cannot be overstated. Allow your friends to show you the love and support they feel for you. Allow them to help you. You and your family have enough to do. Your friends would not ask to help if they were not willing to assist you.

On August 23, 2010, Pat had another PET Scan. The results were sent to Dr. Peters, the chemo oncologist. He suggested that radiation treatments might assure that all cancerous tissues from previous growths were dead. Pat had a consultation appointment with Dr. Emily Militzer, radiation oncologist, to discuss the radiation process and set up the appointment for marking for radiation. That appointment was set for August 27. The morning of August 27, Pat was called and told that the appointment with Dr. Militzer was canceled and that she should go to see Dr. Peters at 3:30 that afternoon. Ken and Pat arrived for the meeting with Dr. Peters and saw him at 5:00 p.m. after his last appointment. Dr. Peters explained that he had made a mistake. He had not seen the second page of the PET scan report. There were two new tumors, one the size of a nickel and other the size of an elongated dime. They were positioned between the kidney and the aorta. Surgery was impossible and radiation was not recommended. How could Dr. Peters have missed that? Does he not read the reports sent to him? Ken was livid. This is an example of where it is important for each patient to have a strong advocate.

> *Suggestion 21: Doctors make mistakes! Let us repeat that. Doctors make mistakes. Where possible, get copies and double check all reports sent to your doctor. Ask questions and get answers. This is where your advocate can be a huge help. Don't assume that the MD behind the doctor's name makes him infallible. Remember, he works for you. Make sure he is doing the job he should be doing. Show him respect always but be tough.*

Pat was so distraught over the news that she might not have been able to ask the right questions and make the right decisions, but having Ken, her advocate, there, was a lifesaver, and that can be taken quite literally. Ken asked a simple question after some discussion. "Dr. Peters, is it time that we considered other hospital options?" Dr. Peters' response was "Perhaps so; I will refer you wherever you want to go." Ken's immediate response, based on his ministry and times of dealing with cancer patients, was "M. D. Anderson, Houston, Texas." Dr. Peters helpfully began the referral process that evening.

> *Suggestion #22: Always have a backup plan if your local medical facility cannot or is not giving you the absolute best treatment. Research cancer hospitals. Find out how they are rated. Are they a cancer research hospital? Are they known to be up to date on all the latest procedures and possible cures? Don't be afraid to ask your doctor for a referral.*

Needless to say, this news was devastating to Pat. Ken could see her distress. He asked Pat, "Do you want me to call Charles?" (their Pastor from First United Methodist Church, Poplar Bluff). Pat said, "Yes." Ken called and only said, "Charles, Pat needs you." His answer, "Ken, I will be there immediately." Twenty minutes later Charles knocked on the door. He spent over an hour with Pat, talking with her and praying with her. Her emotional strength returned and Pat and Ken both made a renewed commitment to beat this no matter what it took.

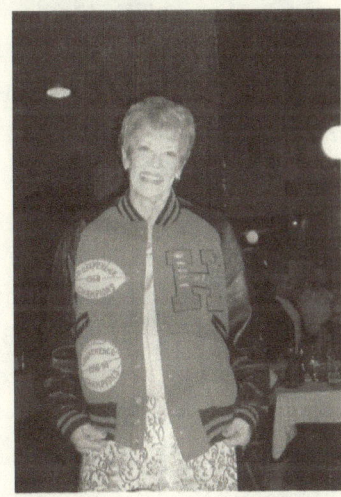

There was an event scheduled for September 11 that Pat had looked forward to for months. It was her Fiftieth Herculaneum, Missouri, High School Reunion. With hope that she would feel well enough to travel and attend, they made the necessary reservations. It was very special for Pat to see friends she had known for fifty years, and it was

Pat at 50th High School Reunion

special for Ken to meet those people. Pat looked well and lovely and as Dr. Peters stated, "If you didn't look so damned good, you'd get more sympathy!"

Suggestion #23: Continue to live your life fully within your physical limits. Visit friends. Go to reunions. Don't immerse yourself so much in your illness that you become a hermit. Have fun!

Dr. Peters' referral to M. D. Anderson was received and Pat was accepted as a patient. M. D. Anderson in Houston, part of the University of Texas Medical System, had been listed by major publications as the number one cancer hospital in the country. The only thing that was disappointing is that Pat's first appointment could not be scheduled until October 25, 2010.

They discussed the trip to Houston and decided that they would combine that trip with side trips to places they would like to visit. The benefits from Pat's Aflac Insurance policy would help make the trip financially possible. They left Poplar Bluff, Missouri, on October 13 and drove to Knoxville, Tennessee, to visit Steve and Rose Anne Bell who had attended their wedding. From there they drove through the Smoky Mountains enjoying the beautiful fall colors. (For those who have not been in the Smokies, the drive from Gatlinburg, Tennessee, to Cherokee, North Carolina, is breathtaking.) They drove across North Carolina to visit Belton and Toni Joyner. Belton had officiated at the wedding. While in the Durham area, they attended the Duke versus University of Miami football game in Wallace Wade Stadium. While there Pat experienced one of the highlights of the trip. Being married to Ken, Pat was "required" to become an avid Duke basketball fan. She had watched every televised game Duke had played the previous national championship season. Her favorite player was Kyle Singler who was named the Most Valuable Player of the

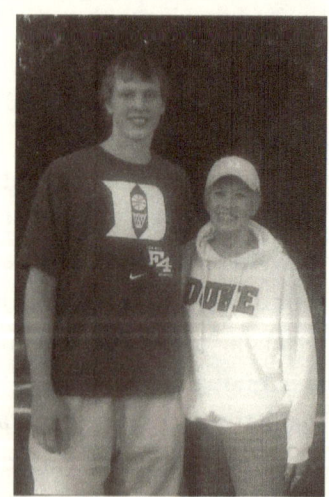

Kyle Singler and Pat

national tournament. While Ken had stepped away, who should come near but Kyle Singler! Belton Joyner took a photograph of Pat and Kyle. Pat prides herself on being 5' 8 ½". And you'd better not forget that ½". Kyle is 6' 8" and Pat felt short for one of the few times in her life. Ken surely regretted that trip to the men's room. It meant that he totally missed meeting Kyle!

They continued to Louisiana where they visited and even stayed at a cottage on the Oak Alley Plantation Grounds, as well as touring the plantation. They then went and toured Nottaway Plantation nearby. Pat's favorite book and movie is *Gone with the Wind* and she often dreams of being the "belle of the plantation." When Ken reminds her that she might have been a sharecropper's daughter, she responds. "It's my dream and I'll be who I want to be, the southern belle."

> *Suggestion #24: Remember that "Bucket List." Cancer insurance money might help make doing those things possible. Seeing friends we rarely visit...check. Driving through the beautiful Smoky Mountains in the fall... check. Going to a Duke football game and introducing Pat to the beautiful Duke campus...check. Meeting Kyle Singler...check. Visiting and spending the night on a southern plantation straight out of "Gone With the Wind"...check. Make the best of your opportunities for travel. Make memories!*

On Saturday, October 22, they arrived in Houston. They wanted to visit a United Methodist church on Sunday so they looked in the telephone book to find one. "Hey, there's one on Main Street and our hotel is on Main Street. That can't be far," Ken stated. They drove and drove and drove to the opposite side of the city. They found the Ebenezer United Methodist Church and entered. The congregation had no problem whatsoever knowing the Birts were visitors. They were the only white faces in the building. The congregation could not have treated Pat and Ken with more love. The members immediately wanted to know the reason for being in Houston and when they heard, they prayed with them for Pat's full recovery. The Birts visited Ebenezer on several subsequent trips to Houston.

Suggestion #25: Practice your faith no matter where you are. God deserves the praise and thanksgiving. He is always there for you!

On Monday, October 25, Pat had blood work done and then all the preparation for yet another CAT scan. Pat is allergic to IVP dye so has to take Benadryl before each scan. After the three hours of preparation and the scan, Pat was loopy. As Ken accompanied her away from the appointment, she was just strolling along, looking at the ceiling, the floor, walls and was totally out of it. A good nap always seems to return her to normal.

On Tuesday morning, they met with Pat's oncologist at M. D. Anderson, Dr. Rachna Shroff. Ken and Pat were both impressed. Dr. Shroff did a full examination of Pat, something that had not been done in the past. She showed the Birts the images of Pat's two growths and then explained how they would be treated. It would require more chemo that could be delivered in Poplar Bluff. The prescription for the chemo "cocktail" would be sent to Dr. Peters and his office would administer it. A copy was also given to Pat. Ken and Pat left feeling that they had indeed found the best. They returned to Poplar Bluff on October 28. Pat's chemo was scheduled to start soon after their return.

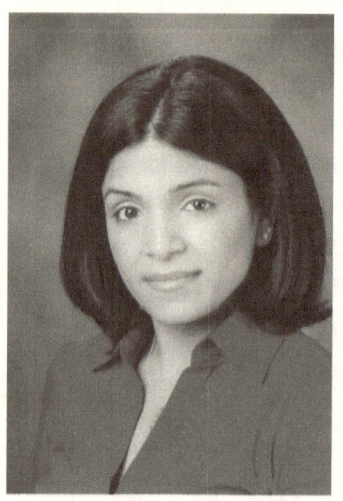

Dr. Rachna Shroff

Suggestion #26: Always, always get a copy of all "orders" from your doctor. The patient will be undergoing the treatments and should be fully aware of the chemo "cocktail" or the treatment to be given. Be prepared to check the prescribed treatment against what was actually administered. Don't be shy. If you don't understand anything, ask! You have a right to this information.

On November 7, 2010, Ken and Pat finally joined First United Methodist Church in Poplar Bluff, having attended there for almost a year. Their Phoenix Sunday School Class came forward and stood with them as they joined.

The first chemo treatment prescribed by M. D. Anderson was delivered correctly. Pat had her usual day or two of discomfort. She was also receiving a shot in her stomach after each treatment to offset the lowering of her platelets. This shot did make her ache all over. That was worse than the nausea that often accompanies the chemo.

On November 15, Pat was scheduled for another treatment. Beforehand, they met with Dr. Peters. He told them that he thought he'd change the prescription for the chemo. He just felt M. D. Anderson was too aggressive. Ken went ballistic asking, "Why are we going to M. D. Anderson if you aren't going to follow their directives?" Dr. Peters somewhat reluctantly said he would administer exactly what M. D. Anderson prescribed. Pat received her treatment. Then, both Ken and Pat began to wonder. Did Dr. Peters do as was agreed upon? Pat, having worked at the hospital, knew a number of people in the pharmacy. She contacted them, showed them her copy of the "cocktail" ingredients and asked for a comparison. Dr. Peters had omitted one ingredient. Ken and Pat were both pretty upset and wrote a letter to Dr. Peters suggesting that it might be time for Pat to work with another oncologist. Dr. Peters felt that the conflict between he and Ken had caused some stress, leading to the doctor's mistake. But, he also knew that the confidence a patient must have in the doctor had been damaged. They still liked Dr. Peters. He is a really great guy and a good doctor, but he was right: patient confidence had been shattered with the two mistakes. They asked for a referral to Dr. Robert Oldham, a colleague in the same office as Dr. Peters. The Birts met with Dr. Oldham, asked him for his guarantee that he'd follow M. D. Anderson's instructions

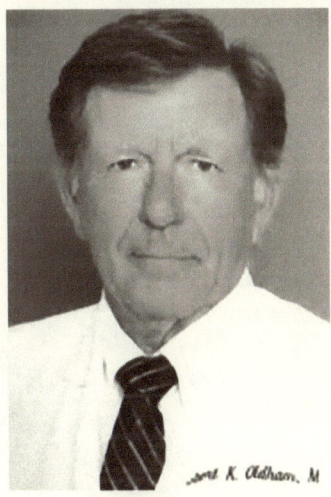

Dr. Robert Oldham

and he readily agreed. In fact, his communication with Dr. Shroff in Houston was frequent and Ken and Pat were very impressed with his care.

> *Suggestion #27: Do not be hesitant about changing doctors. A patient must have full confidence in his/her doctor. Confirm with the new doctor that the cause for the issue will not reoccur. Remember to thank the previous doctor for his/her services. Mistakes do happen. Take the "high road" in your dealings but make the change!*

They were scheduled to return to Houston on December 27, 2010, for the next three month visit. How concerned were they that a cure wouldn't be forthcoming? What legal provisions did they need to make, that everyone should make, whether cancer patient or not?

6

• ◆ •

Time to Make Legal Decisions
– Time to Live Life

E ven though Ken and Pat had every confidence that the cancer could be defeated, they still knew that they needed to be prepared for the worst case scenario. They made an appointment in Poplar Bluff with a lawyer whom Pat had known for years. They saw that powers of attorney were drawn up giving each the ability to make decisions if the other was unable. They also had wills drawn up and notified their children of the decisions. They wanted to make sure that there were no misunderstandings with family members and they knew that each would make the right decisions for the other if and when necessary. Pat had also written instructions as to what she wished for her funeral arrangements. These were hard things to do, but necessary. (Actually, they should be done by all people regardless of health.)

Suggestion #28: Assure that the patient's will and powers of attorney are current. It is also important to have funeral arrangements written and discussed. If possible, it is always a good idea to have these arrangements paid for so that they won't need to be arranged in a time of

even more stress. Make sure that the patient's family members are aware of the details of the will so that no misunderstandings will take place later. These details should be carried out by all persons, cancer patients or not.

Time was drawing near for the December 27 appointment at M. D. Anderson. The Birts, again, wanted to take side trips to see things that neither had seen before. On December 13, they drove south.

A number of years earlier, Pat had worked in Florida for two brothers, Garfield and Dean Beckstead. The men had together founded Palm Island Resort, located on a barrier island off of the west coast of Florida. Pat had talked to Dean, and Ken and Pat were invited to come to Palm Island, stay in a condo there and just relax for a week. This offer was too good to pass up. It would give both an opportunity to put some of the stress and strain on hold.

They arrived on the mainland near Palm Island on December 15, took the ferry across to the island, were given a golf cart for transportation (since no cars are allowed) and settled into the condo. They had no longer unpacked when the phone rang. It was Dean Beckstead inviting them to meet him and his wife, Jamie, for dinner at the Rum Bay Restaurant that he owned on the island. The Birts had a wonderful meal and while there discovered that Dean and Jamie were also United Methodists. They invited Ken and Pat to go to

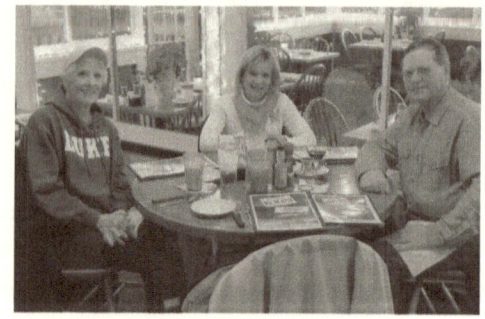

Pat, Jamie and Dean Beckstead
at the Rum Bay Restaurant

church with them on Sunday. They also invited them to a cocktail party at the home of Dean's brother, Garfield Beckstead, who lived in the Oaks, a gated community in Osprey, Florida. Afterward, all would go to the Oaks Clubhouse for dinner.

Ken had seen the web site for Palm Island and noticed that Palm Island

Resort had a naturalist on staff who knew about the fauna and flora of the island. Ken mentioned to the General Manager that, if possible, he'd enjoy hanging out with the naturalist to learn more about the island. Within an hour of Dean's invitation to dinner, there was a knock on the door. Al Squires, the naturalist, was there with an invitation for a tour of the island the next afternoon, a tour the Birts thoroughly enjoyed.

On Saturday night, Jamie, Dean, Pat and Ken left Palm Island and drove to The Oaks in Osprey, Florida, about an hour away, for the cocktail party at the home of Gar and Sanae Beckstead. A number of people that Pat had known for years were there. Besides the Becksteads, there were Tim and Chris Fitzsimmons (Tim is the General Manager of Useppa Island, a private island owned by Gar Beckstead) and Terry and Barbara Lynch. (Terry is

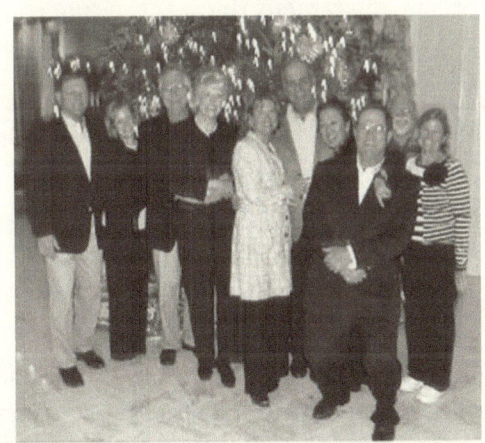

The Group at the Oaks

the owner of Palm Island Marina.) The hors d'oeuvres and cocktails were wonderful. When it was time to go to dinner, Gar came to Pat and Ken and said, "You're riding with Sanae and me." They walked out the front door and there sat a brand new blue and silver Rolls Royce. They rode less than a mile but felt they were in real luxury. Pat admitted later that she slipped her shoes off just to feel the three inch lambs' wool carpeting. Dinner was wonderful and Ken and Pat had no idea at that time what an impact these people would have on their journey. "Friends come second only to God in the love that has been shown to us," Ken said. "We credit them with much of Pat's healing."

The next day, Sunday, they went to church with Dean and Jamie. Pat had worked during the construction of Palm Island Resort (and also Useppa Island) with Dean and Gar Beckstead. There had been great times and there had been rough times. Pat shared with Ken, "I had no idea; if anyone 20 years ago had told me I'd be sitting in a church pew with Dean

Beckstead, I'd have never believed it." After church Ken and Pat took Dean and Jamie out for lunch.

Ken and Pat left Palm Island on December 21 and drove along the coast of Mississippi, stopping at Beauvoir, the after-war home of Jefferson Davis, the President of the Confederacy. They then drove to New Orleans, a city that Pat had never visited. They stayed in the French Quarter at the Prince Conti Hotel. The first stop that night was at Pat O'Briens for dinner and of course, the famous Hurricane, a rum concoction that leaves one reeling. The next day they walked the French Quarter from the hotel down to the Mississippi River front. They had beignets at Café Du Monde and then shopped along the Riverwalk. They stopped at hat shops and Pat looked for the coolest hats she could find. She was rapidly losing her hair and knew she'd use them. On Christmas Eve, they joined a Walking Haunted Tour. It was really cold that night and Pat would have paid anything for a warm scarf. A very nice shop keeper sold her one for half price. (Being cold is one of the negative side effects of chemotherapy.) On that tour, they met a really nice couple, Ron Monk and Alison Monroe. The four became immediate friends. Most restaurants were not serving breakfast on Christmas morning, but The Prince Conti did, so the Birts invited Ron and Alison to join them. Ron and Alison arrived carrying a very large gift bag full of goodies as a Christmas gift. "Where they found all the things in the bag with such short notice we still do not know," Pat mused. After breakfast, the four spent the day at Harrah's Casino, since very little else was open. Christmas night, they enjoyed a light dinner at Ron and Alison's hotel. Again, friends, new or old, are blessings to anyone but even more important for those on the cancer journey.

Pat and Ken left for Houston and M. D. Anderson the next morning with full intentions of returning to New Orleans for New Year's Eve and Day. On December 26, they arrived at the Rotary House International in Houston, the hotel owned by and attached to M. D. Anderson. Pat underwent her blood work and CAT scan on December 27. They were nervous but also anxious to get Dr. Shroff's report on the morning of December 28. Her report was good. Pat's two tumors had shrunk slightly from the chemo treatments, and there were no new growths. Another appointment was set for March, 2011, a year and one month into the journey, with more to go.

During the trip to Houston, Ken and Pat had decided not to go back home via New Orleans. The attitude was one of "seen it, done it." They canceled their reservations and started for Missouri. It was wise that they did that because both returned home with a viral infection. It was better to be sick at home than hundreds of miles away.

7

Hair by Chemo and Now Radiation

After Ken and Pat returned to Poplar Bluff, life returned to normal. Chemo under Dr. Oldham continued every two weeks. Pat had plenty of opportunity to wear her new hats bought in New Orleans. She was losing hair more rapidly. She was given wigs by UCAN (United Cancer Assistance Network) in Poplar Bluff. Most people who saw Pat didn't even know that she was wearing a wig. But, Pat made the decision to shave all her hair off. She got tired of hair on her pillowcase and getting into her mouth. This was done in January, 2011. This decision was the correct one but still was one

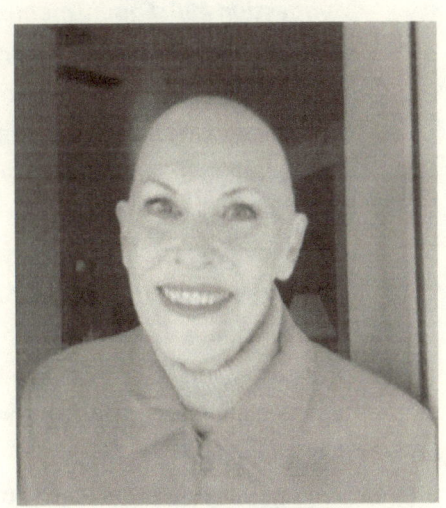

Pat with Hair by Chemo

of the few times Pat shed tears. In jest, one of Pat's sons said, "Mom, your hair will grow back; mine won't!"

Suggestion #29: When cancer patients lose their hair, it is very, very traumatic, often leading to tears and depression. Friends and family need to be aware and supportive during this time.

Ken and Pat continued their activity in the church and especially enjoyed Pastor Buck's friendship and the support of the Phoenix Sunday School Class. On the Birts' return from Houston, the class never failed to applaud as they came into the classroom. Ken began to meet for breakfast on Tuesday mornings with Dan Barbour, a member of the class and a psychologist at Kneibert Clinic. What many people don't realize is that caregivers are the forgotten victims of cancer. Ken needed someone with whom to talk, someone with whom to seek counsel. Dan provided this and the meetings meant a great deal to Ken. For even more fellowship, Ken also investigated joining the Lions Club and attended a number of meetings.

Suggestion #30: Family members and friends should stay in touch with the patient's caregiver. The responsibilities of the caregiver are exhausting, sometimes physically, but always emotionally. Caregivers, find a close friend or counselor with whom you can share. Also, get involved in an activity or two that takes you away from the house and the responsibility. A friend or family member will be glad to stay with the patient if necessary.

Pat and Ken made their third trip to M. D. Anderson in March, 2011, with no side trips. Pat went through her normal blood tests and CAT scan on March 1. They again stayed at the Rotary House International. It was very convenient because there were skyway bridges straight from the hotel to the hospital. Ken and Pat remained amazed at the size of M. D. Anderson. It is made up of numerous buildings. And the elevators are lettered from A through Z and then from AA and up. But, the signage is great and if one ever needs help, there is someone right there not only to give directions but to take one to where one needs to go. Ken had been in dozens of hospitals in his years of ministry. Never had he seen service like this. One is treated as a guest, rather than a patient or family member. One thing they did notice on all their trips to Houston: Cancer is no respecter of age, sex or nationality. They met people from all over the world who had come to Anderson for treatment. On one occasion they saw a group that turned out to be a sheik followed by his several wives all dressed from head to foot in black with faces partially covered. One could only imagine how uncomfortable the women must have been particularly in the Texas summers. However, the group, being from a Middle Eastern country, may not have felt the discomfort that Ken and Pat would have felt.

On March 2, they had a meeting with Dr. Shroff. The two tumors had

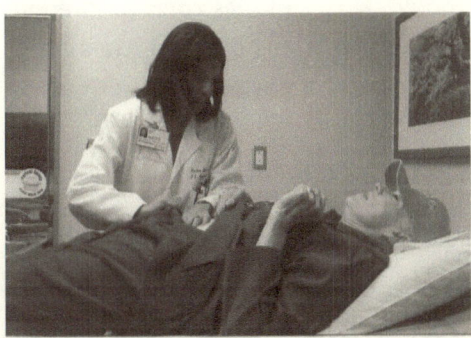

shrunk even more and there were no new growths. Dr. Shroff continued Pat on che-motherapy to be delivered by Dr. Oldham in Poplar Bluff and with instructions to re-turn again in May, 2011. They made the two day drive back to Poplar Bluff.

Dr. Shroff Examines Pat

Ken, as a caregiver of a cancer patient, knows the stress that caregivers go through. It's not only the constant care that must be provided, taking patients to their doctor's appointments, sitting through hours of chemo or radiation therapy, taking over some of the household chores the patient is no longer able to do, but also the stress of just worrying about a loved one. For this reason, he made the decision to start a Cancer Caregivers Support Group. First United Methodist Church in Poplar Bluff volunteered the space and support for the meetings. Knowing that it might not be possible for a caregiver to leave a patient, the decision was made to have a Cancer Patient Support Group meet at the same time. Ken led the Caregiver's Group and Pat led the Patient's Group. *The SEMO Times*, a weekly Poplar Bluff newspaper, published an article to promote the groups. The reporter who wrote the article interviewed oncologists, as well as others involved in Pat's case. Both patient and caregiver definitely need a support group.

Suggestion # 31: If there is not a cancer or caregiver support group in your area, think about spearheading the effort to start one. Churches and hospitals are often willing to help.

In May, 2011, the Birts again returned to Houston and M. D. Anderson with no side trips. Again, Pat went through the blood work and the CAT scan. Again, they met with Dr. Shroff. Dr. Shroff was pleased that the two tumors had shrunk a little more and that there were no new growths, but she had a concern. Pat's platelets were low. Platelets are minute bodies found in the blood plasma that function to promote blood clotting. The chemo was taking a toll on her body. Dr. Shroff was concerned about prescribing any more chemo. That was the status of future treatments when Ken and Pat left Houston. They were depressed and didn't know what the future held.

In the hotel that night, the phone rang. It was Dr. Shroff. She said, "Pat, I took the liberty to send your records to a radiation oncologist here at M. D. Anderson, a man for whom I have the greatest of respect. He studied your records, looked at the images of your tumors. It's true that they are too close to the aorta for surgery but he says he is sure he can kill them with radiation. The techniques are so much better now than they were years ago. I have the greatest faith in this oncologist. What do you want to do?"

Pat burst into tears. Kill the tumors? A chance to be cancer free? Yes, Yes, Yes!

Dr. Shroff told the couple they needed to make plans to return to Houston within the next couple of weeks and plan on staying for over six weeks. All radiation would be delivered at M. D. Anderson.

Dr. Shroff could have simply said, "No more chemo. We'll think about where we go from here." But, she didn't. She took the initiative to contact the radiation oncologist immediately. Having Dr. Shroff as Pat's doctor at M. D. Anderson was added to the list of God's blessings and miracles.

Needless to say, the Birts returned to Poplar Bluff and began making plans for a six week trip to Houston. Where would they live? M. D. Anderson supplied a list of hotels and apartments. Going online, the Birts found the list, and began to make decisions. A hotel was just out of the question. The daily rate might be in the family budget but there would be the cost of meals and parking at the hospital. Then, they discovered the Esplanade Apartments. They could get a fully furnished one bedroom apartment for $80 a day. It included indoor secure parking and a shuttle service to and from M. D. Anderson. Thanks to the wisdom of Pat's having kept her Aflac Cancer Insurance, the policy would pay $60 a day. Plus, Aflac paid a sizable amount for each radiation treatment and Pat would need 29. (Remember, in Chapter 2 where they told the story of how close they had come to letting the Aflac Insurance lapse! It is what they consider a miracle that Ken sat down at that computer that day and found the invoice. Two days later and the insurance would have lapsed.) Without that insurance, M. D. Anderson and what turned into a two months stay in Houston would have not been possible.

We do serve a God of great blessings.

Suggestion #32: If travel to and from treatment is necessary, investigate the possibility of free air travel through the American Red Cross. Often they have volunteer pilots who provide this service. Also contact your hospital for suggestions on discounted hotels or apartments. And if your hospital does not offer that service, don't be hesitant to ask the hotel or apartment if there are special rates for patients and their families. Most establishments will offer a discount.

8

Houston, It's a Go!

Pat and Ken arrived at the Esplanade Apartments on May 21 with the first appointment with Dr. Prajnan Das, the radiation oncologist, scheduled for Monday, May 23. The Birts met with Dr. Das and were very impressed. He reported that it would take about two weeks for him to complete his work necessary to determine the treatments needed. Pat and Ken had the option of going back to Missouri and then returning to Houston or staying at the Esplanade during that time. The decision was made to stay in Houston since the apartment was already secured and they were settled.

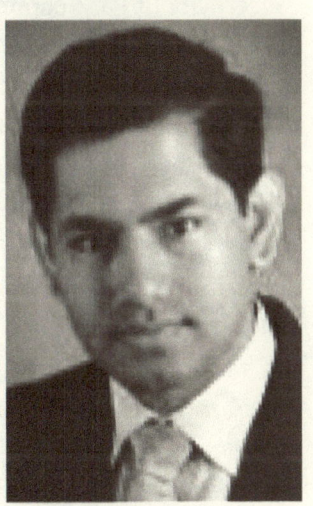

Dr. Prajnan Das

During the waiting period, Ken and Pat enjoyed seeing many of the sights in Houston, as well as taking a side trip to San Antonio, Texas. Ken and Pat had visited San Antonio previously and were very impressed with the city, particularly the River Walk. The weather on the previous trip was perfect and the sightseeing was very enjoyable. However, this trip in the month of June was a different experience. The hotel Pat and

Ken had chosen was only blocks from the River Walk. They strolled to Landry's Restaurant for a very nice seafood dinner. However, the weather was unbearably hot. Pat and Ken were both feeling the discomfort. They began the walk back to the hotel. Although it was only five or six blocks, Pat had to stop numerous times to rest from the heat. Ken admitted that the heat was too much for him as well. It is important that caregivers be very careful to assure the patient does not suffer from too much heat or too much cold. When feeling well, both tend to forget that the patient's body is very susceptible to both. *(See Suggestion #13.)* The following morning Ken approached Pat about leaving San Antonio a day earlier than planned. Pat readily agreed. The Birts decided to drive to an area about an hour west and visit the Natural Bridge Wildlife Ranch. This trip proved to be well worth the additional miles. After visiting the park, Ken and Pat, unable to find a hotel, drove back to Houston that evening.

The Esplanade Apartments were within walking distance of several museums, as well as the beautiful Hermann Park. Free concerts were held in an outdoor theater at the park and Pat and Ken enjoyed one of the evening offerings. Since it is warm in Houston in May, Ken had some concern about Pat's comfort at the concert. They were prepared to take a small ice chest with drinks and then decided to wet towels and keep them in the ice chest for cooling their faces. Ken got the idea of freezing the cloths before putting them into the chest. This extra step proved to be appreciated as the evening was very warm. Life's joys can still be found in uncertain times.

Several days prior to the first scheduled radiation treatment, Pat was tattooed to mark the targeted area. The tattoos were only small dots and were the first tattoos Pat had ever received. She commented, "How can anyone stand being tattooed? Just the placement of the dots stung like crazy!" Pat was also fitted for the mold in which she would lie while receiving the treatments. She also learned that it would be necessary for her to take three Xeloda chemo capsules every morning and every evening for the six weeks of treatment. Fortunately, this very expensive medication was covered entirely by M. D. Anderson and Pat's insurance. Pat also learned she would need to receive 29 radiation treatments, one a day, Monday through Friday for six weeks.

On Monday, June 13, 2011, the treatments began. Throughout the day, a shuttle bus operated from the Esplanade to the hospital. Passes could be purchased at the apartment office. On days when only a radiation treatment was required, free parking was also provided by the hospital. On Fridays, when, in addition to the treatment, Pat saw Dr. Das, (and the visit would be over two hours), Ken and Pat rode the shuttle.

Pat's treatments were administered by a wonderful group of technicians. Ken remained in the waiting area where magazines, puzzles and even refreshments were available. A treatment took less than 30 minutes and was scheduled in the morning, leaving the remainder of the day free for Pat to rest or for the Birts to do more sightseeing.

While waiting for the shuttle one day, Pat and Ken met another couple, Corey and Cindy Knapp from Albuquerque, New Mexico. Corey was a patient requiring a bone marrow transplant from his brother. Corey's immunity was compromised and he had to be very careful about infections. The Birts have stayed in contact with the Knapps since and Corey is recovering nicely, but they still make their periodic trips to M. D. Anderson for follow-up examinations.

> *Suggestion #33: Be aware that a patient's immune system will be compromised. Be cautious of crowds, hospitals and other places where harmful germs might be lurking. Caregivers who are sick and patients should consider wearing a mask.*

On July 27, 2011, Pat had her last radiation treatment. This was a very special day! As is the tradition at M. D. Anderson, she rang the bell that signifies the end of treatments. Ken and Pat couldn't begin to say how much they appreciate the care given by Dr. Das

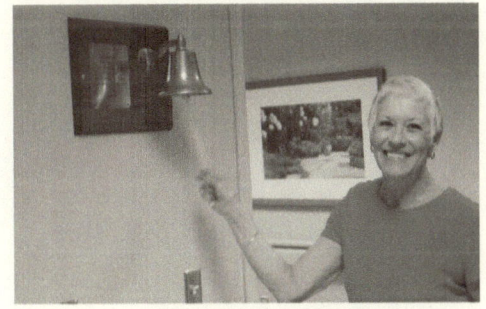

Pat Rings the Bell

and the radiation technicians, Claudia, Travis and Joann among others.

Suggestion #34: Remember to celebrate the major and minor events in your cancer journey. Also remember to thank the medical personnel who have been part of each step of the journey. Your thanks does much to underline the very reason they chose their lifework. Celebrate! The very act itself aids in the miraculous healing process.

It would be necessary for Pat and Ken to return to M. D. Anderson in three months in order to find out the results of the radiation treatments. The appointment was set for October 10, 2010. That date couldn't come soon enough for them.

The next day, Thursday, July 28, Ken and Pat, left to return to Poplar Bluff not knowing what life-changing events awaited them there.

9

◦ ◆ ◦

A New Home in Paradise

Ken and Pat knew that they would not be staying in Poplar Bluff another year and their lease on the duplex expired on August 15. The Birts had never felt "at home" in the duplex. Their landlord sometimes seemed to be overly protective of his property and there was very little privacy for Ken and Pat. The landlord's home was on a hill that overlooked the duplex and his actions were too invasive and at times, felt rude. Ken knew that the landlord wanted another full year's lease so on the way from Houston to Poplar Bluff, the Birts talked about what they would do.

Sure enough, upon their return, the landlord called and wanted to talk about renewal of the lease. Ken and Pat decided that they'd offer the landlord a guaranteed 90 day lease and that if they left before the expiration of the 90 days, they would still pay the full rent for that period of time. What if the landlord would not accept this offer? To work an alternative plan, Pat called Gar Beckstead, a friend who lived in Osprey, Florida. She knew he also had a plantation home in Alabama as well as homes in Florida. She asked Gar about the two areas. It was important for Pat to live in an area that was warmer than Missouri. In her conversation with Gar, he offered for Ken and Pat to come to Alabama to stay at his plantation and look over the Talladega area. He did caution, however, that Alabama could be cold in January and February. So, as an additional offer, he suggested the Birts come to Osprey, near Sarasota, and stay in his guest condo at the Oaks Club, a residential community, where one of his homes was located. They could look over that area for a suitable place to live. With these offers in pocket, they awaited the landlord's visit.

As the Birts had expected, the landlord was resolute that they sign a full year's lease. Ken and Pat gave notice that they'd vacate the duplex prior to August 15 when the lease expired.

> **Suggestion #35: Sometimes it is necessary to make difficult decisions during your journey. Something within us says, "Don't do it. Hang with the known." But, those going through the journey should make the decisions that will be best for them. God opens the necessary doors. Let your "gut" lead you. It is rarely wrong!**

Immediately, Ken began making phone calls. First, he called the landlord and announced their plans. Ken and Pat then called Gar and accepted his gracious invitation to stay at his guest condo in Osprey and let him know they'd arrive in less than a week. Ken then called a moving company and arranged for the packing of the duplex and the loading of the truck prior to August 15. The Birts then called a friend to come and oversee packing and loading. Pat then called her good friend, Dana Beckwith, who had taken care of their feline son, Sam, when they were in Houston. Pat asked if Dana would come and clean the duplex so that their landlord would have no complaints. All was arranged. Several days after this, Ken and Pat packed the two cars, including Sam, to begin the journey to Florida. They were again the receivers of help of wonderful friends and a very gracious God.

On July 27, Ken and Pat drove away from Poplar Bluff, Missouri. They stopped for the night in Atlanta for a short visit with Alan Galumbeck, the best man in their wedding. Sam had travelled well. He had settled on the floorboard of the back seat and never moved on the first ten-hour day and the second eight-hour day. What a good traveler!

On the afternoon of Thursday, July 28, Ken and Pat arrived in Osprey, Florida at the guest condo and moved in. Kathy, Pat's daughter, and her husband, Mike, met them upon arrival and took Sam since Ken and Pat did not feel the cat should be in the guest condo. Kathy is a lover of cats and the Birts knew that Sam would be well taken care of.

> *Suggestion #36: Friends and family are part of God's greatest gift. Let them know what they can do to help when you are in need.*

The following morning, Friday, the Birts were invited to the Beckstead's home a few blocks away for coffee with Gar and Sanae, his wife. After spending time with them, Ken and Pat launched a quest for a new home.

They began to search north of Sarasota in Bradenton, Florida, then traveling 58 miles south to Port Charlotte, Florida. They had decided to rent an apartment and had sold most of the items that they wouldn't need: lawnmowers, lawn implements and gas grill. They looked all day Friday and Saturday. They found nothing that they thought they would be happy living in. On Sunday, they went out again and were once more disappointed. After lunch on Sunday, they decided to stop and buy a newspaper. Thinking perhaps they might rent a house instead of an apartment, they looked at the ads in the newspaper. At a convenience store where they stopped to buy a paper, Pat picked up a free community paper. Returning to the guest condo, they began to look through the rental ads.

They looked through the daily paper first not finding anything that looked as if it would meet their needs. Then, Ken picked up the free community paper. Immediately he saw a house for rent in Venice, Florida. Again, God guided us via a newspaper! The rent was equal or less than the apartments being considered. The phone number was out of state; Ken called. Jim Sadler answered. He owned the house in Venice although he lived in Rochester, Minnesota. Ken told him of their interest. Jim gave the Birts the address of the house and said he could probably arrange for a realtor to meet Ken and Pat and open the house for them to see on Monday.

> *Suggestion #37: Coincidence? Luck? Fate? A miracle? When good comes your way, regardless of what you call it, stop and thank your God for His blessings. He opens*

***doors for you over and over again if you are just open
to His urgings. We were, and we were blessed over and
over. Remember to thank Him!***

Excited about the prospects of finding a home, Pat and Ken got in the
car that Sunday evening and drove to the address Jim had given them. The
house was on a cul-de-sac in a lovely community. The house sat on a
beautiful lake and had a large lanai stretching the full width of the house.
The main doors were locked but the lanai was open. They walked around
the yard, looked at the lake and entered the lanai. They could see very
little of the inside of the house but decided, "We will make this work
regardless of what the condition of the inside." They called Jim so he could
arrange for the realtor to show them the inside.

On Monday, they met the realtor and she took them through the
house. Although the yard and inside of the house needed loving care,
they knew it was for right for them. There was even a large walk-in closet
for Pat. The walk-in closet was a big selling point. The house had three
bedrooms, a large living room and dining room and a small TV room. The
kitchen was equipped with very nice appliances. The house needed a

lot of work on the floors and
the walls, and the carpet was
filthy. But, they knew they
could bring the inside and
outside up to high standards.
They called Jim and told him
they wanted the house. They
said, "We will treat the house
like we own it and if we ever
leave, we'll leave it in better

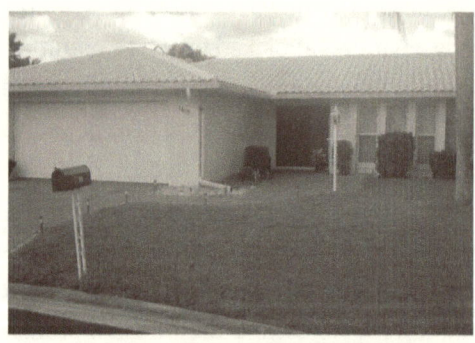

Our New Home in Venice, Florida

condition than we found it." Jim wanted an eighteen month lease to which
they readily agreed. The realtor gave them a key immediately. This was
August 5. They called the movers and arranged for delivery on August
17. The duplex in Poplar Bluff would be vacated prior to the August 15
deadline. They also called friends in Poplar Bluff to confirm the packing and
loading dates, as well as arranging the date for the duplex to be cleaned.

Little did they know that the landlord in Poplar Bluff would withhold from the deposit a large amount for not giving him a full 30 days notice of cancellation of the lease, as well as other charges they did not feel they should pay. But, they were finished with him as a landlord and just felt relief. Jim Sadler, the owner of their new home, turned out to be the perfect landlord, paying for any repairs or major maintenance. He arranged for a workman to come in and do touch up painting, cleaning and hanging of curtains. Jim was just happy to have good renters that would care for his investment.

Having keys to the new home gave the Birts almost two weeks to work in the yard and in the house to ready it for the delivery of their furniture. Of course, they had to buy a lawnmower, gas grill, plus other yard appliances they would need.

On August 17, the furniture arrived and within a week they were totally settled in their new home. Their neighbors on the cul-de-sac were wonderful and really were thrilled that the Birts' home was being kept up and was so beautiful. Ken and Pat thought, "We are now Floridians."

What would they do to find a local oncologist in Venice? How would their next visit to M. D. Anderson turn out? Were the radiation treatments successful? They still had a two month wait to find out.

10

•◆•

Good News and Now a
Honeymoon Cruise

P at and Ken's move to Venice, Florida, was well-timed. Pat's oncologist
  in Poplar Bluff, Dr. Robert Oldham, had accepted a position as the
Director of Oncology at a hospital in Key West, Florida. Now, in Venice,
Pat would have to find another doctor to coordinate care with Dr. Shroff
in Houston. As a past hospital employee, Pat knew that most hospitals
have a directory of all physicians who practice with them. She secured
the directory for Venice Regional Medical Center. In that resource she
could see a picture of doctors, read their credentials including the medical
school they attended and their years of experience. Pat chose Dr. James
Rubinsak and met with him on September 16.

> *Suggestion #38: When looking for any doctor, check with
> your local hospital and get a copy of their directory of
> doctors. Read their credentials. You can also research
> the doctor on the Internet and often learn more about
> him/her.*

Dr. Rubinsak's office was under five minutes from the Birts' new

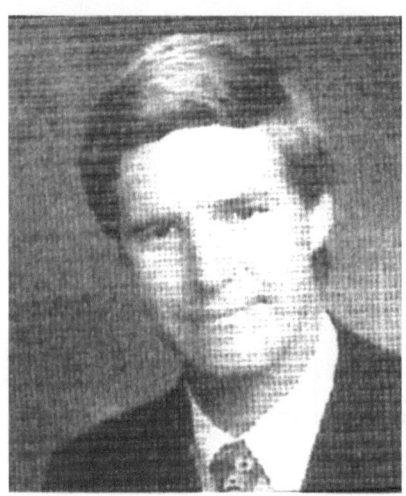

Dr. James Rubinsak

home. It was necessary for Pat to have her port flushed once a month as well as having blood work done to check her low platelets. She immediately found Dr. Rubinsak to be an excellent doctor.

As mentioned earlier in the book, Ken and Pat were good friends with Dr. Belton Joyner and his wife,Toni. Belton had performed Pat and Ken's wedding ceremony. Toni had been ill for some time requiring several hospitalizations. After a number of unsuccessful procedures, Toni passed away on Wednesday, September 21. Ken and Pat left immediately for North Carolina to be of any possible help or support for Belton and to attend the visitation and funeral. Ken was asked to be a pall bearer. The Joyners had been married for almost 52 years and the loss was very difficult for Belton. Making the loss even more difficult, the funeral was held on Belton's 76th birthday. Pat and Ken did all they could to undergird Belton at this time of loss. They stayed in the area several days before returning home.

> **Suggestion #39: As you go through your own journey, remember that other people are also on journeys. Be available, as possible, to others who are in need and offer them your love as you also assure them of God's love.**

Upon their return to Venice, Pat and Ken began to plan their next trip to Houston and M. D. Anderson. They would leave on October 7 and stay at the Rotary House International, owned by M. D. Anderson. The Rotary House was a hotel, managed by Marriott, connected to the hospital by two skywalks and very convenient. The Birts could park their car and not move it until they left Houston if they so chose. Restaurants were available in the hotel as well as the hospital. The drive to Houston was longer from Florida, than from Missouri, so Ken made reservations for Daphne, Alabama, approximately halfway. Pat was feeling good and the trips, though tiring, were enjoyable for her and for Ken.

Two forms of entertainment were planned for the long drives. First, Ken and Pat would rent CD's and listen to books on the trips. They also enjoy crossword puzzles. Ken is a visual person and this allowed him to participate even when driving. Pat would read a clue from a puzzle and together they would find the words.

> *Suggestion #40: Make your driving trips fun. Make frequent stops at interesting places. Listen to books on tape. Go to the Internet and find games for trips, particularly if children are involved. Watch license plates and make a list of every state you see. Have fun!*

Pat and Ken arrived in Houston on October 8 and checked in at the Rotary House. Pat's appointment for her blood work and CAT Scan was on Sunday, October 9. Sunday arrived and Ken and Pat crossed the skywalk for her appointments. All went well except for the fact that Pat was just as loopy from taking the Benadryl as always. But, a nap and a good meal perked her up.

Pat's appointment with Dr. Shroff was Monday morning. This was the appointment the Birts had been looking forward to for three months. Had the radiation been effective? Of course, Ken and Pat were both nervous. They were not really scared because they had always felt that God was with them and He would see them through whatever the outcome. But, they were certainly nervous.

The report was good. The growths had not metastasized to any other part of Pat's body. In fact, the two growths had actually reduced in size, something that does not usually happen under radiation. Dr. Shroff was surprised and pleased as were Pat and Ken. Of course, another appointment at M. D. Anderson would be necessary in three months, and Pat would still see Dr. Rubinsak in Venice every month for a port flush and to have blood work done.

Ken and Pat began the trip back to Venice immediately after the appointment with Dr. Shroff, stopping again for the night in Daphne, Alabama. They arrived safely at home on October 11.

Suggestion #41: Remember to give God the praise for safe travels.

Since moving to Venice, Ken and Pat had been visiting Grace United Methodist Church. The pastor of Grace, the Reverend Tom Derrough, had been very welcoming and the Birts soon attended a New Member's Class to learn more about the church. They had also become active in the Christian Encounters Sunday School Class where Ken taught occasionally. On October 23, they became members of Grace.

Pat was feeling so well that the Birts decided that they could schedule their honeymoon cruise that they had cancelled in May. They decided on a ten day cruise, December 8 through 18, to the Caribbean on *The Emerald Princess.* Pat and Ken had saved every penny they received in wedding gifts, for birthdays and Christmas as well as all coins they collected in a bank. They wanted to enjoy the cruise with no new debt. They met some really nice people on the ship and visited the islands of St. Kitts, St. Lucia, Barbados, Antigua, St. Thomas and Princess Cays. All went well until two days before the cruise ended. Ken contracted a virus and had to visit the ship's infirmary. Pat

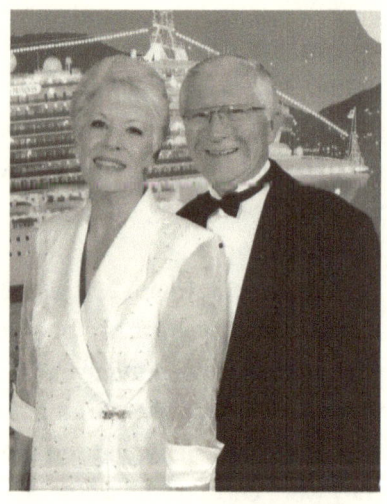
Pat and Ken on the Cruise

was well until the last day when she also came down with the virus. Upon landing in Ft. Lauderdale, Pat shared with Ken that she had been coughing up blood. Ken and Pat were both frightened over this occurrence. Ken began the three hour trip back to Venice and drove straight to the Venice hospital's Emergency Room. Knowing Pat's cancer history, the attendants took her straight in and began tests. After several hours, including blood work and a CAT Scan, Pat was released and the problem was diagnosed as the viral infection. Pat and Ken were so relieved. They could now go home and unpack and rest from just too much fun.

> *Suggestion #42: In the event that the cancer patient suffers anything physical that would be out of the ordinary, don't hesitate to have it diagnosed. It might not be critical but finding out relieves stress the patient, caregiver and family don't need to be under.*

When Pat and Ken moved to Florida, they were told that they'd have a lot of visitors who would love to leave their cold climates in the north for a visit to the sunny state. Invitations to visit went out to friends and relatives. Did friends respond? Well, of course they did!

11

Medical Appointments Can Go Awry

Visitors did schedule times to come to Florida. But before the visits began, Pat and Ken had to return to Houston for Pat's January, 2012, visit. They left Venice on January 6 stopping for the night in Daphne, Alabama, again. By now, the hotel desk clerks knew the Birts on sight. They traveled on the following day to The Rotary House International and Pat's appointment. Her blood work and CAT Scan were done on Sunday, January, 8, with her appointment with Dr. Shroff scheduled for Monday morning. Of all the trips to Houston, this one was the most disappointing. Because of the demolition of an M. D. Anderson building a block from the main hospital, everything was in a state of caution. No one could get to the hospital via the skywalk until shortly before appointments on Sunday. Then, when Pat did arrive for her CAT Scan, she went to the room where the procedure was to be performed. Upon entering the CAT Scan area, she saw the technician in a rather amorous embrace with another employee. The staff, perhaps these two, had also left out one procedure vital to having a CAT Scan. When Pat was given a blanket for warmth, the technician told her she'd have to hold her arms up over her head instead of having them under the blanket. In jest, Pat said, "Can't I leave them here where it's warm?" He responded rather rudely, "Well, it's either stay warm or cancer!" Pat was rather shocked by his response.

The following day, instead of meeting with Dr. Shroff, Pat and Ken met with her Physician Assistant. The assistant told Pat that the two tumors had reduced further and that there were no new growths. Pat and Ken left the hospital and started the drive back to Venice. The farther they drove the more frustrated they became. First, there was the lack of professionalism on the part of the CAT Scan technician. They were disappointed after making the two-day trip that they did not see Dr. Shroff.

They arrived back at home on January 11. They were still very disappointed in their treatment at Anderson. Pat sat down and wrote an e-mail to Dr. Shroff's nursing assistant, not the PA who had met with us. At 9 AM the next morning the Birts' phone rang. It was Dr. Shroff. She apologized to them and told them that she had had every intention on meeting with them, but that the PA had not told them to wait and they were gone when Dr. Shroff went to meet with them. She also said that she would contact the necessary people about the unprofessional behavior of the technician. The Birts regained their full confidence in Dr. Shroff and M. D. Anderson. Ken and Pat asked themselves, "How many doctors would personally call the patient and apologize?" They were again impressed.

> **Suggestion #43: If you are ever disappointed in the service provided by your doctor or the hospital, let your disappointment be known. They will never know a problem exists if not told. Most hospitals will appreciate your notifying them and will respond.**

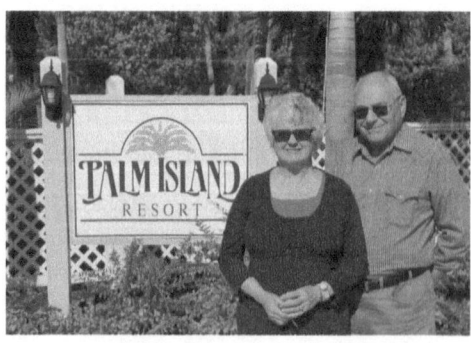

Rose Anne and Steve Bell

The time to entertain our visitors had arrived. Steve and Rose Anne Bell (who had been members of Ken's church in Oak Ridge, Tennessee) came to visit on January 13. Steve and Rose Anne had driven from Oak Ridge for the Birts' wedding and have been wonderful friends. Ken and Pat took them to dinner at Sharkey's, a favorite seafood restaurant on Venice Beach. They also took the Bells to Palm Island where Rose Anne found numerous beautiful shells. The visit was great.

On January 17, Belton arrived for a week's visit. They showed him all the sights, including a day's trip to Useppa Island and a day at Palm Island. They all took in the Ringling Museum in Sarasota, as well as a number of good restaurants. This visit was the first vacation Belton had had in years and he thoroughly enjoyed it as much as Ken and Pat enjoyed having him visit.

In late 2011, Ken had been introduced to Useppa

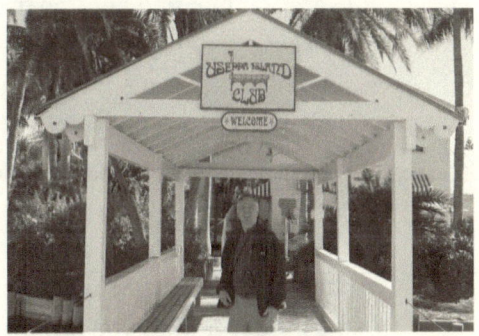

Belton on Useppa Island

Island lying off the west coast of Florida. The Birts' friends, Gar and Sanae Beckstead, own the private island. When Pat suggested they go visit Useppa Ken was not as excited as Pat was. Ken had spent a week on Palm Island and thought Useppa couldn't possibly be as nice. The day the Birts arrived on Useppa, it was cold and raining. Ken wasn't impressed. He even told Pat, "I think I like Palm Island more." The following day, the sun was out and it was beautiful. Transportation was a golf cart provided for us and they began to explore the island. Ken had never seen anything as beautiful. Useppa even had a small museum covering the island's ten thousand years of habitation. Bones of Calusa Indians dating back six thousand years had even been found. Ken was blown away. It was and is a magical place.

Upon returning to Venice, Ken made a major decision. He wanted to write a book on the ten thousand year history of Useppa. He asked Gar Beckstead's permission and Gar promised him full access to the island and his full cooperation. Ken began writing. As of this date, the book has fourteen chapters and is within a month of submitting for publication. The magic of Useppa has fully instilled itself in Ken and Pat.

Archaeology has been a big part of Useppa's history. In order to better understand archaeological digs, Ken requested permission to participate in a dig scheduled for March 12 through 24. Permission was granted. Gar invited Pat and Ken to stay in Gasparilla Cottage, the Beckstead home on Useppa. Ken and Pat spent every day the first week digging, sifting and finding fascinating artifacts. Pat was feeling well enough that she outworked Ken on the dig. The second week, Pat worked all day several days while Ken worked on his book which he had entitled *Useppa, An Ongoing Journey*. Ken and Pat met and became friends with Dr. Bill Marquardt and Dr. Karen Walker, archaelogists from the Museum of Natural History at the University of Florida. The Birts also met a number of the residents on Useppa and made some friends for life. Those friends have continued to support the Birts on their cancer journey.

> **Suggestion #44: Never allow yourself to get so self-absorbed in your own journey that you stop making friends. Next to God and family, friends are invaluable. They want to share your journey with you, even new ones.**

Time was approaching for Pat's next appointment at M. D. Anderson. What would this visit tell them? Would it be good? Would they see a much longer and more painful journey in front of them? Of course they would be nervous until they met with Dr. Shroff again.

12

—◆—

The Impossible Can Be Possible

The date of Pat's next appointment at M. D. Anderson quickly approached. Ken and Pat were concerned that the news might not be as good as it had been at the last visit. Pat had been as well as she had ever been. But, the insidious cancer might have metastasized again in a new location. Ken assured Pat that everything would be great. The Birts discussed asking about transferring Pat's care to Dr. Rubinsak and Venice Regional Medical Center because of the long and exhausting drive to and from Houston. But, both Pat and Ken agreed that they wanted Dr. Shroff to continue to oversee Pat's care. They left Venice on April 6, 2012, for Pat's scheduled appointments beginning Sunday, April 8.

> *Suggestion #45: If you are pleased with the progress of your health under the care of your current oncologist and hospital, don't change. If carrying the financial burden concerns you, talk to the hospital. Often times there are plans that might relieve some of the strain.*

Again, Pat and Ken stayed in Daphne, Alabama, the night of April 7 arriving at the Rotary House International the evening of Saturday, April 8. Pat went through her normal blood tests and CAT Scan, this time with no issues with the technicians. Pat and Ken had a nice dinner at the hotel restaurant and got a good night's sleep. They knew after their appointment with Dr. Shroff they would be starting their long drive home.

Almost immediately after being taken to Dr. Shroff's examination room, the doctor entered with a huge smile on her face and hugs for both Pat and Ken. Was the news good? Definitely! It appeared from all the tests that the two tumors had shriveled up and were most likely dead. In a layperson's terms it appeared that Pat was cancer free. The Birts couldn't believe the wonderful news. Dr. Shroff made two very nice comments. First, she said, "Pat, you make M. D. Anderson look good." Then she added in a hushed voice, "I shouldn't say this but you are one of my favorite patients." Dr. Shroff then shared that she had visited Florida recently and ask herself, "I wonder how close I am to where Pat and Ken live?" She still wanted to continue to see Pat but this time the Birts could wait for six months to return to Houston. Dr. Shroff wanted Pat to see Dr. Rubinsak for blood work and definitely call M. D. Anderson if Pat had any symptoms. Dr. Shroff would stay in contact with Dr. Rubinsak. The Birts again expressed their appreciation to Dr. Shroff and hugs were shared among all three.

Ken and Pat got into the car and began their trip home. Their hearts were the lightest they had been in the 28 months of the journey. As soon as they reached I-10 heading east, they began making phone calls. They called Pat's Mom, Belton Joyner, the Reverend Charles Buck and others. Ken and Pat said, "We were beyond happiness!"

Upon returning home, Ken and Pat made a list of all the doctors and medical personnel who had been so supportive during the journey. They wrote a personal letter to each, saying a very sincere thank you. Pat sent flowers to Dr. Shroff with a big thank you. Dr. Shroff was on her way to the airport when the flowers arrived. Her Administrative Assistant called Dr. Shroff's cell phone and said, "You've got to come back." Dr. Shroff returned and met her assistant at her car. Dr. Shroff was given the flowers. She immediately called Pat to thank her.

> **Suggestion #46: When you get good news, remember first to thank our loving God and then thank those medical professionals who have been given the gifts**

of healing. Doctors are not always thanked for their service. And, stories such as the Birts are the reason they chose the medical field. Thank them!

Not expecting any replies from the letters, Pat was surprised when she received an e-mail from Dr. Griffith's Office Manager, a friend of Pat's from her hospital days, telling Pat how excited Dr. Griffith and the entire staff were to hear the news. How wonderful that they responded! Several days later, the Birts were so pleased to receive a personal, handwritten letter from Dr. Oldham celebrating Pat's news. Pat then received a letter from Dr. Peters, Pat's first oncologist. Not only did he relate the joy he and his staff felt to hear the good news but he said, "My congratulations to M. D. Anderson on their good work." This doctor was the one who thought M. D. Anderson was too aggressive. How surprised and pleased we were with Dr. Peters' note! Two weeks later we received a letter from the head of the Oncology Department at M. D. Anderson, thanking Pat and Ken for their very kind letter. The Birts thought they also needed to write letters to all the family and friends who had been so supportive. Since the beginning of the journey, Ken had been sending updates to a group of friends and relatives updating them on Pat's progress. E-mails poured in from this group with their good wishes.

Pat had one more wonderful piece of news. Her granddaughter, Kristin Kimsey Strohm, gave birth to a healthy baby boy, Remington Allen Strohm. Pat was a great grandmother, a blessing that she might not have experienced had the first prognosis held true.

On June 19, 2012, Pat and Ken celebrated their second wedding anniversary with a wonderful dinner at a Japanese steakhouse, a second anniversary that many thought would never happen due to Pat's health. The day was made even more special when they received an anniversary poem written by their good friend, Belton Joyner. It was so special and so true. They want to share the poem with the readers of this book.

A Poem for Ken and Pat

When love comes to broken places,
When life's pains have left their traces,

Then the joy of new beginnings
Breaks into our underpinnings,
Making us again in wholeness,
Living life again in boldness.

Thank you, God, for healing graces
And tomorrow's life-filled places.

Ken and Pat could not be happier. Pat had begun to paint again. Others say she is a very accomplished acrylic artist. And, they continued working on their two books, *Useppa, An Ongoing Journey* and this book, *A Journey of Love and Miracles*. There was no doubt in Ken's and Pat's minds that they were the children of a loving God, and had a loving family and loving friends. Ken's and Pat's love for each other was itself a gift. And, one might call it coincidence or luck, but both Ken and Pat know that more miracles are occurring in the journey than can be counted. There are no coincidences!

Where does this leave us on our journey? Is it over? What does the future hold?

13

◦━◆━◦

The Journey Continues
but Never Give Up!

I s the journey over for Pat and Ken? No, it continues. Pat needs to continue to monitor her health, with visits to Dr. Rubinsak every three months and to Dr. Shroff at M. D. Anderson every six months. Her cure will never be taken for granted. The insidious destroyer of lives, cancer, could return at any time. But now, knowing that Pat had stage 4 colon cancer and that statistics dictated a life expectancy of a year, Ken and Pat can only thank their God and all the doctors, family and friends who were so instrumental in their journey.

Ken and Pat know that every cancer story doesn't have a happy ending. Statistics state that 570,199 cancer deaths will occur in 2012. Courage through the journey can be a happy story even if the ending is not what we hoped for. The Birts have written this book in the hope that their story about how they lived the journey will be a help to others who are also on the journey. The suggestions are not a cure but hopefully they will help patients, caregivers, families and friends face the journey. It might seem trite to quote the old adage, "God doesn't give you more than your shoulders can carry," but Ken and Pat confirmed that God does love them and displays that love through the doctors, hospitals, relatives and friends in their lives.

Ken and Pat prayers daily are for you, the patient, and you the caregiver, and you the families and friends of the patient. Hang in there! Remember as Jim Valvano said, "Don't give up! Don't ever give up!"

Now, allow Ken and Pat to list below the forty-six suggestions that helped them on their journey. Some of these might seem repetitious. They are! We consider them that important.

Suggestion #1: It is important to tell those closest to you if you experience any discomfort or symptoms of any kind that concern you. Another person, friend or family, can support and perhaps advise you.

Suggestion #2: It is always a good idea when planning a cruise or trip where trip insurance is available to pay the small amount for that. In the event of sickness or emergency, the insurance will save you from the lost investment. We were glad we took cruise insurance.

Suggestion #3: Listen to your inner-self. Sometimes a change of plans might be exactly what God directs. God works in marvelous ways and Ken and Pat believe He does communicate with you and directs you in the correct path.

Suggestion #4: When you experience a continuing health issue that can't be diagnosed, it is time for you to have an advocate with you, a person who will ask the hard questions and make sure the medical personnel use every option at their disposal. In Pat's case, many laypersons would have thought, "Why not a CAT Scan?"

Suggestion #5: Encourage friends and relatives to be positive with the patient. One person needs to be the patient's advocate. That person must be a strong advocate. Having a number of people sharing their cancer stories with the patient can be very disturbing. Friends should do the loving things that friends do, bring dinners, magazines and books, offer to clean the house or run errands. The common statement made by friends is "Let me know if you need anything!" Don't wait to be asked. Just do those small things that will mean so much to the patient and their family.

Suggestion #6: Ken had always thought cancer insurance was a waste of money. Not so! It is a small price to pay for the financial help the insurance can offer. Health Insurance should be kept up to date and should cover prescription costs. But where will the money come from that will pay for costs not covered by health insurance? Aflac is one provider of cancer insurance. There are others. It IS a good investment.

Suggestion #7: In the event that a patient's insurance does not cover a medication, talk to the doctor and his or her staff. They can be of tremendous help and can often find a solution.

Suggestion #8: The patient should have an advocate, usually a family member or a friend. That person should be with the patient on every treatment and every doctor's visit. The advocate can ask the hard questions, ask for an explanation when something is not understood and watch for consistency in the treatments. If a step seems to be left out, the patient or advocate should ask why. Doctors and treatment centers do make mistakes, so ask!

Suggestion #9: If you are a person of faith, make your congregation and especially your pastor, priest or religious leader fully aware of your condition. The pastor will visit, listen and offer prayer. The small groups within the congregation will also bring comfort and offer their help. Accept that help! Make them a part of your team!

Suggestion 10: If the patient or immediate family has a senior parent, assure that person is taken care of and that minimal help will be needed by the patient or his or her immediate family. Make sure the senior parent's affairs are in order in the event of a death or serious illness. The patient and immediate family have a full plate and shouldn't have to worry about caring for an aging parent's affairs. Sometimes the most caring thing is to plan ahead.

Suggestion #11: The caretaker needs to have an outlet for their frustrations, physical and psychological needs. The caretaker is the forgotten victim of cancer. Friends, a minister or a caregiver's group can fill this need. However, if the caregiver leaves the home for any length of time, make sure the patient has the care and support they need in the primary caregiver's absence.

Suggestion #12: Don't postpone major events if the patient is well enough to participate. Allow friends to help with the planning and carrying out the event. Friends want to do this. Let them!

Suggestion 13: Be sure that all precautions are taken if the patient is to be in extreme hot weather. Chemo does impact the body's chemistry. Hats and long sleeves should be worn to fend off the heat and, if necessary, the patient should be settled in as a cool a spot as possible.

Suggestion 14: Continue to live life with all the gusto possible. Everyone has a "bucket list" whether it is written or not. Live life! Start living those dreams from the patient's bucket list. Make memories!

Suggestion #15: Patients, share your down times with your family, your caregiver and your spiritual support person. If you are a private person, get over it! They want to help. Let them do that!

Suggestion #16: Remember, caregivers, family and friends are all under a great amount of stress. Cancer impacts everyone. Be patient with each other. Any serious illness is a time for family togetherness. Be a family. The patients don't need the stress of worrying about those they love battling over their illness.

Suggestion #17: Make sure that all facts related to the patient's employment and insurance coverage are known to family as well as the primary caregiver. Don't be caught unaware that insurance is about to be canceled or that income will cease. Be prepared! Have an insurance agent whom you know well and trust.

Suggestion #18: Can the patient and family care for the home in which the patient lives? Can the family take care of the inside as well as the outside of the house? Is it time to downsize to save labor for the patient and family? These are good questions to ask.

Suggestion #19: Be open to other's offers to help. It's so easy to say, "Thank you, but we have it covered." Even strangers can often help. With security always in mind, allow strangers to become friends. They will be blessed and so will you.

Suggestion #20: This fact cannot be overstated. Allow your friends to show you the love and support they feel for you. Allow them to help you. You and your family have enough to do. Your friends would not ask to help if they were not willing to assist you.

Suggestion 21: Doctors make mistakes! Let us repeat that. Doctors make mistakes. Where possible, get copies and double check all reports sent to your doctor. Ask questions and get answers. This is where your advocate can be a huge help. Don't assume that the MD behind the doctor's name makes him infallible. Remember, he works for you. Make sure he is doing the job he should be doing. Show him respect always but be tough.

Suggestion #22: Always have a backup plan if your local medical facility cannot or is not giving you the absolute best treatment. Research cancer hospitals. Find out how they are rated. Are they a cancer research hospital? Are they known to be up to date on all the latest procedures and possible cures? Don't be afraid to ask your doctor for a referral.

Suggestion #23: Continue to live your life fully within your physical limits. Visit friends. Go to reunions. Don't immerse yourself so much in your illness that you become a hermit. Have fun!

Suggestion #24: Remember that "Bucket List." Cancer insurance money might help make doing those things possible. Make the best of your opportunities for travel. Make memories!

Suggestion #25: Practice your faith no matter where you are. God deserves the praise and thanksgiving. He is always there for you!

Suggestion #26: Always, always get a copy of all "orders" from your doctor. The patient will be undergoing the treatments and should be fully aware of the chemo "cocktail" or the treatment to be given. Be prepared to check the prescribed treatment against what was actually administered. Don't be shy. If you don't understand anything, ask! You have a right to this information.

Suggestion #27: Do not be hesitant about changing doctors. A patient must have full confidence in his/her doctor. Confirm with the new doctor that the cause for the issue will not reoccur. Remember to thank the previous doctor for his/her services. Mistakes do happen. Take the "high road" in your dealings but make the change!

Suggestion #28: Assure that the patient's will and powers of attorney are current. It is also important to have funeral arrangements written and discussed. If possible, it is always a good idea to have these arrangements paid for so that they won't need to be arranged in a time of even more stress. Make sure that the patient's family members are aware of the details of the will so that no misunderstandings will take place later. These details should be carried out by all persons, cancer patients or not.

Suggestion #29: When cancer patients lose their hair, it is very, very traumatic, often leading to tears and depression. Friends and family need to be aware and supportive during this time.

Suggestion #30: Family members and friends should stay in touch with the patient's caregiver. The responsibilities of the caregiver are exhausting, sometimes physically, but always emotionally. Caregivers, find a close friend or counselor with whom you can share. Also, get involved in an activity or two that takes you away from the house and the responsibility. A friend or family member will be glad to stay with the patient if necessary.

Suggestion # 31: If there is not a cancer or caregiver support group in your area, think about spearheading the effort to start one. Churches and hospitals are often willing to help.

Suggestion #32: If travel to and from treatment is necessary, investigate the possibility of free air travel through the American Red Cross. Often they have volunteer pilots who provide this service. Also contact your hospital for suggestions on discounted hotels or apartments. And if your hospital does not offer that service, don't be hesitant to ask the hotel or apartment if there are special rates for patients and their families. Most establishments will offer a discount.

Suggestion #33: Be aware that a patient's immune system will be compromised. Be cautious of crowds, hospitals and other places where harmful germs might be lurking. Caregivers who are sick and patients should consider wearing a mask.

Suggestion #34: Remember to celebrate the major and minor events in your cancer journey. Also remember to thank the medical personnel who have been part of each step of the journey. Your thanks does much to underline the very reason they chose their lifework. Celebrate! The very act itself aids in the miraculous healing process.

Suggestion #35: Sometimes it is necessary to make difficult decisions during your journey. Something within us says, "Don't do it. Hang with the known." But, those going through the journey should make the decisions that will be best for them. God opens the necessary doors. Let your "gut" lead you. It is rarely wrong!

Suggestion #36: Friends and family are part of God's greatest gift. Let them know what they can do to help when you are in need.

Suggestion #37: Coincidence? Luck? Fate? A miracle? When good comes your way, regardless of what you call it, stop and thank your God for His blessings. He opens doors for you over and over again if you are just open to His urgings. We were, and we were blessed over and over. Remember to thank Him!

Suggestion #38: When looking for any doctor, check with your local hospital and get a copy of their directory of doctors. Read their credentials. You can also research the doctor on the Internet and often learn more about him/her.

Suggestion #39: As you go through your own journey, remember that other people are also on journeys. Be available, as possible, to others who are in need and offer them your love as you also assure them of God's love.

Suggestion #40: Make your driving trips fun. Make frequent stops at interesting places. Listen to books on tape. Go to the Internet and find games for trips, particularly if children are involved. Watch license plates and make a list of every state you see. Have fun!

Suggestion #41: Remember to give God the praise for safe travels.

Suggestion #42: In the event that the cancer patient suffers anything physical that would be out of the ordinary, don't hesitate to have it diagnosed. It might not be critical but finding out relieves stress the patient, caregiver and family don't need to be under.

Suggestion #43: If you are ever disappointed in the service provided by your doctor or the hospital, let your disappointment be known. They will never know a problem exists if not told. Most hospitals will appreciate your notifying them and will respond.

Suggestion #44: Never allow yourself to get so self-absorbed in your own journey that you stop making friends. Next to God and family, friends are invaluable. They want to share your journey with you, even new ones.

Suggestion #45: If you are pleased with the progress of your health under the care of your current Oncologist and hospital, don't change. If carrying the financial burden concerns you, talk to the hospital. Often times there are plans that might relieve some of the strain.

Suggestion #46: When you get good news, remember first to thank our loving God and then thank those medical professionals who have been given the gifts of healing. Doctors are not always thanked for their service. And, stories such as the Birts are the reason they chose the medical field. Thank them!

Ken and Pat thank you for your interest in this book. They hope that it helps whether you are a patient, caregiver, family member or friend. You are taking a journey that millions of people take annually. Know that you are not alone. All journeys do not progress as positively as Ken and Pat's journey has progressed thus far, but NEVER GIVE UP! NEVER, NEVER GIVE UP!